Fourth Edition

Tell Me What to Eat If I Have Diabetes

Nutrition You Can Live With

Elaine Magee, MPH, RD

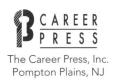

CAREER
PRESS

The Career Press, Inc.
Pompton Plains, NJ

TELL ME WHAT TO EAT IF I HAVE DIABETES, FOURTH EDITION
EDITED BY ROGER SHEETY
COVER DESIGN BY: LUCIA ROSSMAN/DIGI DOG DESIGN
Printed in the U.S.A.

To order this title, please call toll-free 1-800-CAREER-1 (NJ and Canada: 201-848-0310) to order using VISA or MasterCard, or for further information on books from Career Press.

The Career Press, Inc.
220 West Parkway, Unit 12
Pompton Plains, NJ 07444
www.careerpress.com
www.newpagebooks.com

Library of Congress Cataloging-in-Publication Data
Magee, Elaine.
  Tell me what to eat if I have diabetes : nutrition you can live
with / by Elaine Magee, MPH, RD. -- Fourth edition.
        pages cm
  Includes index.
      ISBN   978-1-60163-306-4   --   ISBN   978-1-60163-486-3   (ebook)
      1. Non-insulin-dependent diabetes--Diet therapy. I. Title.

RC662.18.M34 2014
616.4'6240654--dc23

                                                                2013040939

This Anniversary Edition is for the 26 million people in the United States with diabetes and the estimated 79 million American adults with pre-diabetes.

Contents

Introduction

There are 26 million people in the United States with diabetes and an estimated 79 million American adults with pre-diabetes. This diagnosis isn't the end—it can be the beginning of your new journey into a higher level of health. You may not have chosen this disease, but where you go from here is indeed your choice. It is my sincere hope this book helps you travel down a healthier and happier path.

If you've just been told you have diabetes, I hope you will find comfort in knowing that there has never been a better time than now to start managing and improving your diabetes. Researchers know more today than they did just five years ago about diet, insulin, other medications, complications, and more!

Let me tell you about what I call the "Diabetes Double Whammy" that comes from modern-day living. Insulin-resistant type 2 diabetes can be traced to the obesity epidemic that arose after World War II. The responsibility of making food for the family started shifting from the family kitchen to factories and restaurants, which tended to make high-fat and sugar, calorie-dense foods. On a large scale, people started consuming more calories on a daily basis at the same time that fewer calories were being burned in this modern-day, technological age. The obvious solution to the Diabetes Double Whammy is moving food preparation back to the family kitchen as often as possible and staying physically active to increase the number of calories burned, in spite of living in this high-tech age.

Three known factors that increase the risk of type 2 diabetes are obesity, age, and lack of exercise. You can't do anything about age, but you can change the other two risk factors, obesity and exercise. In terms of dietary changes, the truth is that it would have been much easier to write this book if there was one specific diet to recommend for all persons with type 2 diabetes. But there isn't. All persons with type 2 diabetes are not created equal. Each person needs to work out his or her particular eating, exercise, or medication plan so that it translates into normal blood sugar in his or her particular body. Some people seem to have better blood sugar with meals low in fat, whereas others do better with meals richer in monounsaturated fat, in which 30 to 40 percent of calories come from fat. But no matter which type of person you are, you will still need the tools to make better meal choices and balance carbohydrates, fat, and fiber in your meal plan. I'll give you those tools. There are other food patterns and nutrients that seem to help most people with diabetes. I'll talk about those too.

Most diabetes specialists believe there are four keys to managing diabetes:

1. Monitoring your blood glucose levels.
2. Exercising regularly.
3. Wise meal planning.
4. Medication and prescriptions.

This book, *Tell Me What to Eat If I Have Diabetes, Fourth Edition*, will obviously spend the bulk of its pages on the third key. But don't be surprised if you find some tips on the first two as well. As a matter of fact, exercising regularly and monitoring your blood glucose are two of the 10 Food Steps to Freedom in Chapter 4.

I also wanted to reintroduce my other book to you, *Food Synergy*, which is about how components within whole foods, and between different foods, work together in your body for maximum health benefits. For example, these are the possible foods or food partnerships with the type of synergy that might improve blood sugar control: fiber, whole grains, soluble fiber in oats, beans, and ground flaxseed. The following are foods with synergy that seem to help keep insulin levels steady: whole grains, soluble fiber in oats, soy protein, and ground flaxseed.

I hope, as you read *Tell Me What to Eat If I Have Diabetes, Fourth Edition*, you will feel as though I am holding your hand and walking with you as you begin this journey. I know how difficult, and sometimes depressing, having type 2 diabetes can be. I held my dad's hand through the last 20 years of having this disease. He wasn't very interested in helping his body live longer and better with diabetes. But, hopefully, you are. I wrote this book to help *you*.

The best gift I can give you is to help you feel great and get your diabetes under good control, all while eating foods you love and enjoy. This book will get you closer to that goal. That is my promise.

Publisher's Note

This book is not intended as a substitute for medical advice. Readers are encouraged to consult with a doctor before following this or any other dietary device.

Chapter 1

The Who, What, Where, Why, and How of Type 2 Diabetes

Diabetes is reaching epidemic proportions. It is the third or seventh leading cause of death in the United States, depending on whether you include the people with diabetes who die from related cardiovascular disease. Roughly 26 million Americans already have diabetes and many more will get it in the coming years as baby boomers age and the rise in adult and child obesity continues. Experts say that about eight to nine million Americans are totally unaware they even have diabetes. Often, they don't find out until fairly severe damage has been done to their bodies. What kind of damage? Uncontrolled diabetes is the leading cause of blindness, kidney failure, and leg amputations. But a wise diabetes educator once told me that "controlled" diabetes is the leading cause of…nothing! That's the truth and the good news.

Once you have diabetes, your risk for heart disease can be four times greater. So telling you what to eat for type 2 diabetes also has to include telling you what to eat to reduce your risk of heart disease. In fact, the types of food and meal choices that work best for diabetics (lower sugar, lower sodium, high fiber, lean meats and plant protein, fruits, and vegetables, with sources of monounsaturated fats and omega-3 fatty acids) are great for someone *without* diabetes who is just trying to eat right and prevent disease. The only difference is that someone *with* diabetes needs to carefully control and monitor his or her blood sugar and, therefore, sometimes needs to keep count of carbohydrate, fiber, and fat grams throughout his or her day.

? What is insulin, and what does it normally do in the body?

Insulin is a hormone normally produced as needed by the pancreas, and one of its major jobs is helping get glucose (energy) into various body cells. When blood glucose levels rise, the pancreas makes more insulin and releases it into the bloodstream. The insulin then causes body cells to remove the excess glucose that is circulating in the blood. In the liver and skeletal muscle cells, the insulin encourages the production of glycogen (the storage form of glucose). In the liver and fat cells, insulin encourages fat production (stored energy). At the same time, insulin discourages the breakdown of body fat for energy (lipolysis), causing the body to rely more heavily on the recently ingested carbohydrates for current energy needs.

? What is type 2 diabetes?

Type 2 diabetes is a metabolic disorder resulting from the body's inability to make enough or properly use insulin. As discussed, insulin is a hormone that triggers body cells to convert sugar, starches, and other foods into energy. Type 2 diabetes is a result of insulin resistance and can occur when the body produces plenty of insulin, but the insulin cannot do its job. For some reason, the cells in the body have become resistant to insulin. In most cases, being overweight or obese for a period of time brings on the insulin resistance, but there are people who are obese for many years who never develop diabetes. So scientists suspect that some people have a genetic predisposition, that their particular genes make them more likely to develop type 2 diabetes under certain conditions, such as aging, weight gain, or an inactive lifestyle. About 90 to 95 percent of people with diabetes have type 2.

? What are the warning signs of type 2 diabetes?

Some people with type 2 don't have obvious signs, but they could have any of the following symptoms:

- Frequent infections.
- Blurred vision.
- Cuts that are slow to heal.
- Tingling and/or numbness in hands or feet.
- Unusual thirst.
- Frequent urination.

- Extreme hunger.
- Unusual weight loss.
- Extreme fatigue.
- Irritability.

? Why do some people get type 2 diabetes?

Insulin resistance is the common cause, but not all people with type 2 diabetes are created equal. Most people with type 2 diabetes start with the potential to develop the disease, such as a genetic predisposition based on family history or ethnicity, which eventually becomes manifested through environmental factors such as aging, weight gain, or a sedentary lifestyle, all leading to insulin resistance.

? Can changing my lifestyle improve my type 2 diabetes?

In the past five to 10 years, important studies have been published documenting how good exercise is for people with diabetes or at risk for developing it. The National Institute for Health did a study to find out whether the onset of diabetes in a high-risk group could actually be prevented. They compared a lifestyle modification program that included healthy changes including nutrition, exercise and a minimal amount of weight loss (Hello! This is the Elaine Magee way of living!) with a treatment program that relied on medication. Guess what happened? The lifestyle program ended up trumping the treatment program! The lifestyle program was twice as good, twice as powerful, with an almost 60 percent reduction in the onset of diabetes, compared with those using medications, which reduced it by 30 percent.

All in favor of working out today and enjoying a nice high-fiber dinner with smart fats featured, say aye!

? Is type 2 diabetes an outcome of nurture or nature?

Behavior, rather than genetics, may provide the key to reducing a woman's risk of developing type 2 diabetes. Results from the Nurses' Health Study suggest that the majority—an estimated nine out of 10 cases—of type 2 diabetes could be prevented by weight loss, regular physical activity, healthy diet, absti-nence from smoking, and moderate consumption of alcohol (half to one drink per day for women). The risk reduction was similar for women with and without a family history of the disease. Because diabetes is a major risk factor for cardiovas-cular disease, such modifications may help prevent heart disease. Researchers fol-lowing nearly 85,000 nurses for 16 years concluded that an estimated 91 percent of the 3,300 new cases of type 2 diabetes diagnosed during the study could have been prevented by lifestyle modifications.

Excess body fat was the single most important risk factor in the development of type 2 diabetes. The heavier a woman was, the greater her risk of developing the disease, even if she was at the high end of a normal BMI (body mass index, a measure of body fat). An estimated 97 million Americans are overweight or obese, making them all at an increased risk for diabetes.

Lack of physical activity was also a significant risk factor, independent of body weight. Conversely, women who exercised seven or more hours weekly cut their risk by 50 percent, compared with sedentary women. About 75 percent of the U.S. popu-lation is considered to be minimally engaged in physical activity or daily exercise.

The women at lowest risk ate a diet high in cereal fiber and polyunsaturated fats, and low in saturated and trans fat. They abstained from smoking and drank moderately (*Nurses' Health Study* 9 [2002]).

? What are the end points of uncontrolled diabetes?

Uncontrolled diabetes is the leading cause of blindness in working-age adults in the United States, accounting for 24,000 new cases of blindness every year. The National Eye Institute estimates that 90 percent of lost vision is preventable. Uncontrolled diabetes is the leading cause of end-stage renal disease in the United States. Approximately 28,000 patients with diabetes develop end-stage renal disease every year. With all the current therapies now available, future cases of end-stage renal disease are probably preventable. Uncontrolled diabetes is the leading cause of non-traumatic lower extremity amputations in the United States. Keep in mind that about 95 percent are thought to be preventable, another incentive to manage your diabetes well!

? How will this book help?

I know it takes some time to really accept that you now have diabetes. This may take a few months or a few years, depending on the person.

A good friend of mine was in what you could call "diabetic denial" for about two years—not exercising, not really paying attention to her blood glucose or what she ate. She was one of the first people to whom I gave a copy of the first edition of this book. Every time I would see her, I would ask if she had read it. She would always have an excuse.

Finally one day she said, "I guess I better start acting like a diabetic." Almost overnight she started monitoring her blood glucose; counting carbohydrates, fat, and fiber; and working some exercise into her busy work week. She feels much better now. Guess what? She had finally read the book.

If you are reading this book right now, chances are you have accepted that diabetes is now a part of your life. You want to make it work for you. You want to manage your blood glucose, reduce your risk of heart disease, and just plain feel better. Because you *want* to make changes, this book can help.

? How do I get my type 2 diabetes under control?

Many diabetes specialists believe there are four keys to diabetes management success:

1. Monitoring blood glucose levels.

You need to monitor your blood glucose, because that's how you know right away if you are keeping it near normal. And you need to keep your blood glucose near normal if you want to protect your body from developing diabetic complications further down the line. If your healthcare team knows how your blood sugar is being affected from day to day, they can help fine-tune your medications, your eating plan, and your exercise routine.

Measuring your blood glucose will tell you rather quickly whether your treatments (diet, exercise, and pharmacological) are working for you. Make sure someone on your healthcare team clearly demonstrates how to measure your glucose and how to record it so it can be referred to easily at follow-up visits.

This is very important in the management of diabetes. Next to the discovery of insulin, the ability to monitor blood sugar was the biggest breakthrough in the treatment of diabetes.

The American Diabetes Association recommends a goal of 90 to 130 milligrams per deciliter (mg/dL) for preprandial (pre-meal) blood glucose levels in adults with diabetes. The American Association of Clinical Endocrinologists recommends that adults aim for a preprandial blood glucose goal of less than and equal to 110 mg/dL.

Generally, blood glucose levels are taken two hours after a meal, which is thought to be when the blood glucose concentrations are at their peak. The American Diabetes Association recommends less than 180 mg/dL for peak postprandial (post-meal) glucose levels. The American Association of Clinical Endocrinologists recommends adults aim for a postprandial goal of less than or equal to 140 mg/dL.

Hemoglobin A1c levels are directly related to blood glucose concentrations over the previous two to three months. The A1c test is often given twice each year in stable patients and four or more times a year in patients for which glycemic control is more challenging. The A1c test goal is less than or equal to seven percent. The following table shows the mean blood glucose levels that correlate with various Hemoglobin A1c test results:

Hemoglobin A1c	Mean Blood Glucose
6 percent	135 mg/dL
7 percent	170 mg/dL
8 percent	205 mg/dL
9 percent	240 mg/dL
10 percent	275 mg/dL

2. Exercising regularly.

Exercise can actually help control blood glucose levels. Exercise depresses insulin production and also prompts skeletal muscle cells to take in more glucose from the bloodstream. With more glucose in your muscle cells, you can produce more energy so that your muscles can continue to work.

Besides helping to control blood glucose levels, exercise improves the cardiovascular system, thus reducing the risk of heart disease, and also encourages weight loss, which can have big benefits for people with diabetes.

3. Planning your meals wisely.

This is the key that this book will give you the most help with. It will help you follow a plan that keeps your personal blood glucose levels normal, protects against heart disease and weight gain, and doesn't make you feel deprived. This book, though, is not about telling you the one and only way to eat; no one diet is best for all people with diabetes. Every person has different risk factors (obesity, hypertension, high triglycerides, kidney dialysis, and so on.) that need to be considered. I will tell you generally which foods or meals are more likely to cause higher blood sugar. But when it comes right down to it, every person is affected by the same food or meal a little differently. Chalk it up to unexplained individual differences.

Generally, many people with diabetes seem to tolerate a more moderate-carbohydrate (around 45 percent of calories from carbohydrate), moderate-fat (around 35 percent of calories from fat) way of eating. Of course, this eating plan requires using mostly canola oil, extra virgin olive oil, avocado, and nuts and seeds, which are high in more desirable poly and monounsaturated fats. Having a couple servings of fish, which is rich in omega-3 fatty acids, each week wouldn't hurt either.

4. Work with your doctor and dietitian on medications and prescriptions specific to your medical condition.

It's important to work with your healthcare team particularly if insulin is part of your treatment plan.

Is there such a thing as too much insulin when it comes to managing or treating type 2 diabetes? Some researchers believe that giving more insulin can lead to increased body fat, as they discussed in a March 2008 press release at UT Southwestern Medical Center. Because high doses of insulin may lower glucose levels, it will also increase the fatty molecules and may cause organ damage, according to new research. Dr. Roger Unger, professor of Internal Medicine at UT Southwestern Medical Center, now believes, after investigating diabetes, obesity, and insulin resistance for more than 50 years, that intensive insulin therapy may not be best for obese patients with insulin-resistant type 2 diabetes, because it increases the fatty acids that cause diabetes. The most rational therapy, he suggests, eliminates excess calories, thereby reducing the amount of insulin in the blood and the synthesis of the fatty acids stimulated by the high insulin levels.

According to Unger, one treatment option to be considered before giving insulin is bariatric surgery. For many with type 2 diabetes, the excess body fat is causing insulin resistance and killing the insulin-producing beta cells in the pancreas. The aim, then, is to correct the insulin resistance by reducing body fat. So it's quite possible that for overweight patients with poorly controlled, insulin-resistant type 2 diabetes, weight loss and major lifestyle changes may actually be more effective than intensive insulin therapy.

But this remains a hot issue among diabetes researchers, so stay tuned, because Chinese researchers have reported that when intensive insulin therapy was given to people just diagnosed with type 2 diabetes, it seemed to improve B-cell (the cells in the pancreas that produce insulin) function compared to using oral hypoglycemic agents.

❓ Where can I go for more information?

To find a Certified Diabetes Educator (CDE) in your area (many provide individual consultations and some offer classes for diabetics), go to *www.diabeteseducator.org*.

For a list of registered dietitians with expertise in diabetes (RD, CDE) in your area, contact the American Dietetic Association's National Center for Nutrition and Dietetics at 800-366-1655 or visit its Website at *www.eatright.org*.

The American Diabetes Association maintains a hotline at 800-DIABETES (800-342-2383), and information on types of diabetes is available by mail, fax, and staff members. The association's Website is *www.diabetes.org*.

Hopefully, your local diabetes center or clinic has a referral sheet available, filled with local numbers for everything from diabetes support groups and counselors to dietitians, diabetes educators, fitness clubs, and personal trainers. If they don't, find somewhere that does. Many hospitals have diabetes support groups, and that is a great starting place.

Chapter 2
Top 3 Profiles of Type 2 Diabetes

I know you may feel as though you have been wearing the label "type 2 diabetes" lately and that health professionals and other people like to lump all type 2s together. The truth is that people with type 2 diabetes come in different shapes and sizes and with different health risks and medical problems. Your health risks and medical problems, in addition to having type 2 diabetes, also define what needs to be done food-wise to help you feel better and live longer. It is important we get these other issues on the table so that you can get a better idea of what your personal diet and food priorities are and how your type 2 diabetes might differ from that of others.

There are certain profiles that stand out in people with type 2 diabetes. I will discuss a few in this chapter. See if any resonate with you.

1. Waiting to lose weight

The good news is that losing weight greatly decreases your risk for type 2 diabetes and can help bring your blood sugar under control if you already have type 2. The challenging part is actually losing the weight and then keeping it off. Let me first say, you are not alone. I understand how difficult it is. I know that, often, thin people actually eat more and exercise less than thicker people. I know what it is like to eat healthy and mindfully, exercise every day, and still not lose weight.

I knew the majority of Americans are considered overweight. But what shocked me was that survey data by the National Center for Health Statistics in 1988–1991 showed a dramatic increase of about eight pounds in mean body weight of American adults since the last survey was conducted (1976–1980). It didn't matter which gender, age, or cultural group you looked at—weight gain still followed.

How can this be? Atkins, Jenny Craig, Weight Watchers, Slim Fast, and other billion-dollar dieting giants have made it their business to wage war against weight gain for decades!

As you've probably heard, one of the first questions related to weight control asks whether the "calories in" equal the "calories out." That's because the net effect of excess calories (more than our current body needs), even in the form of protein, is going to increase the amount of fat put into storage (body fat). We know that most Americans haven't exactly been increasing their "calories out" side of the equation. Due to a combination of modern-life factors (television, long commutes, computers, and so on.), Americans have become more sedentary.

What about the "calories in" portion? True, the average person ate less fat as a percentage of total calories during the survey period (down from 36 to 34 percent), but the amount of total daily calories went up an average of 231 calories compared to 1976–1980. Now we're getting to the real million-dollar question: why would Americans suddenly increase their total daily calories at a time when the country has never been more obsessed with dieting and more concerned about healthy eating?

Maybe because a large chunk of the American population is actively dieting at any one time, they continue to ride the unfortunate weight roller coaster of strict dieting and obsession—deprivation, bingeing and guilt, strict dieting and obsession—over and over again. Studies show that when people diet, the vast majority of them eventually gain the weight back—and then some. Maybe some of these eight pounds are the "and then some" from a country that chronically diets.

Three myths and three facts about obesity and weight loss

Losing weight gradually, not skipping breakfast, eating more fruits and vegetables—these are all commonly endorsed strategies for weight loss and, though they may make good sense, many have not actually been proven, according to researchers from five universities. Don't get me wrong; these sensible strategies may work well as part of a comprehensive weight loss plan/program, but apparently not necessarily by themselves. The other point to consider is that it is inordinately difficult to confirm these associations with randomized studies and observations, as associations related to obesity and weight loss are often complicated by all sorts of factors and variables.

You can find the complete article by this group of researchers in the *New England Journal of Medicine* (2013, 368:446–454), but I've listed three of the most noteworthy myths and facts for you here.

Three myths

Myth #1: Small sustained changes in energy intake or expenditure will result in large weight changes over time.

You often hear weight loss tips such as, just adding 10 minutes of walking a day or drinking one less soda a day will contribute to a certain amount of weight loss. It doesn't necessarily work, nor does the other way around necessarily work either. For instance, eating two extra potato chips will not always contribute to weight gain. But this doesn't consider the diverse aspects of energy balance and how the human body seems to naturally compensate for changes in intake or expenditure. Individual strategies like eating more vegetables or eating breakfast are likely to help only if there is an overall reduction in daily calories, explain the researchers.

The 50-year-old calculation that equates one pound of weight loss to a deficit of 3500 calories came from short-term experiments (generally tested in men on diets with less than 800 calories a day) and isn't accurate for small changes over long periods of time, according to the researchers.

Myth #2: Setting realistic goals in obesity treatment is important because, otherwise, patients will become frustrated and lose less weight.

This sounds reasonable for sure but research hasn't shown consistent negative outcomes when dieters have more ambitious goals. In fact, several studies have shown the opposite: more ambitious goals were sometimes associated with better weight-loss outcomes.

Myth #3: Significant, rapid weight loss is associated with poorer long-term weight loss compared with slow, gradual weight loss.

When rapid weight loss (achieved with very low-energy diets with less than 800 calories a day) was compared with slower weight loss (achieved with diets with 800 to 1200 calories per day) in randomized controlled trials, although the rapid weight loss diets showed more weight loss in the short term, there was no significant difference between the two types of weight loss in the long term.

Three facts

Fact #1: Diets (reducing energy intake, often dramatically, for a period of time) do promote weight loss, but trying to go on a diet or recommending that someone go on a diet generally does not work well in the long term. Obesity is a chronic condition, requiring ongoing management to maintain long-term weight loss. That's probably why short-term diets have abysmal success rates of maintained weight loss at three or five years.

Fact #2: For overweight children, programs that involve the parents and the home setting promote greater weight loss or maintenance. In this way families are attempting to change the lifestyle and environment that potentially encouraged the excessive weight to begin with. Or, looking at it the other way, continuation of the conditions that promote weight loss promotes maintenance of the lower weight.

Fact #3: Physical activity or exercise in a sufficient dose aids in long-term weight maintenance. The best part to me is that even without any weight loss, exercise offers a way to lessen the health-damaging effects of obesity.

The bottom line is that there isn't a one-size-fits-all, magical way to lose weight and keep it off. The issues of obesity and weight gain cannot be attributed to one isolated food or beverage. Just because you see a headline in the news, doesn't make it scientifically proven or applicable to you. Go beyond the headlines and check for yourself, as, often, more research is needed. Talk to your doctor and dietitian and have them customize weight-loss recommendations and help you make the lifestyle change priorities that will most likely work best for you.

The energy balance barrier and how to get around it

If you feel like your body is working against you to lose weight or keep it off, you aren't crazy. Our modern-day environment plus the human body's energy balance regulatory system create the perfect storm for obesity. Knowing how to best weather the storm can be vital to people with pre-diabetes or type 2 diabetes. The good news is researchers know more now about the importance of energy balance to the human body and how we might better trick the body into losing and maintaining weight.

Here are some energy balance basics before we go on. When the body is in energy balance, body weight is stable. Humans take in energy (calories) by consuming food and drink, and expend energy or burn calories through the resting metabolic rate—RMR—(the amount of calories needed to maintain normal body functions), and the thermic effect of food (the amount of calories needed to digest, absorb, and metabolize food/drink), which accounts for about 10 percent of daily energy expenditure. Lastly, of course, is the physical activity throughout the day. The RMR is proportional mainly to lean body mass. Your metabolic rate decreases as you age mainly due to declining lean body mass, which is why it's especially helpful for people over age 50 to do muscle strength and resistance training.

Here are some nuggets of wisdom from a recent report ("The Importance of Energy Balance," *US Endocrinology*, 2013, by James O. Hill, PhD, Holly R. Wyatt, MD, and John C. Peters, PhD):

This is what makes weight loss tricky. Energy input and expenditure are interdependent and regulated at several levels and, as a result of this physiological control, compensatory changes kick in when intake and expenditure change.

Example #1 of how the body compensates: When calorie intake is reduced, the body compensates by stimulating hunger and reducing RMR so less energy is expended. Some bodies, due to their genetic wiring for survival, are better at reducing RMR than others.

Example #2 of how the body compensates: An increase of energy expenditure (due to an increase in exercise) stimulates increased hunger or decreases physical activity at other times of the day.

Guess which end of the energy balance compensation is stronger? It appears that the body's natural compensatory response and changes, when there are fewer calories coming in than being burned, are stronger than when we are taking in more calories than we are burning. This was, of course, good for the survival of the species back in the time of long winters and potato famines, but not so good in modern times. We live in an environment where excess calorie intake is highly likely, while burning fewer calories is also likely due to cars, computers, appliances, televisions, and so on. This helps explain why many people eventually end up in the "obesity" group if their lifestyle hasn't changed. Small, consistent, positive energy balance results in gradual weight gain over time.

Prevention of weight gain is easier than treatment of obesity (although knowing this isn't going to help you if you are already obese).

Think small! Weight loss requires major behavioral changes which trigger compensatory decreases in energy expenditure that then encourage weight re-gain. So think *small*—smaller behavioral changes help trick the body because smaller changes produce less compensation by the energy balance regulatory system. This is a better approach, not only from a physiological perspective but also a psychological one, which is less likely to promote eating disorders and food or body image issues. Prospective studies have shown that small changes in diet and lifestyle can result in lasting weight loss.

100 might be the magic number. It has been estimated that the small changes in energy intake and expenditure totaling 100 calories per day could stop weight gain in most people. This could be simple changes such as:

- Taking the stairs.
- Talking a 15-minute walk after lunch or dinner.
- Switching to diet soda or unsweetened tea once a day.
- Paying attention to eating when you are truly hungry and stopping when you are comfortably full, especially at times when you tend to overeat (like in restaurants).

- Enjoying one scoop of ice cream instead of two (served in a mini cup with a mini spoon so you are more likely to slow down and enjoy the serving).
- Ordering a skinny latte at the coffee house (no whip, made with low-fat or skim milk and possibly sugar-free syrup) or a regular coffee instead of fancy coffee.

Exercise is your secret weapon! Given how the body naturally compensates for changes in energy balance, many researchers suspect that energy balance is easier to achieve at high levels of energy expenditure. In the 1950s, for example, studies reported that energy intake was better matched to energy expenditure when people were physically active. In rat studies, matching energy intake and expenditure was inaccurate at low or high levels of physical activity. Likewise, in human studies, food intake does not seem to drop when energy demand drops. Multiple studies report that, over time, a high level of physical activity is associated with less weight gain whereas lower levels are associated with greater weight gain.

Fad or restrictive diets are helping to fuel the obesity epidemic. Diets and plans promoting food restrictions tend to cause compensatory decreases in energy expenditure and increases in hunger. Many people who do lose substantial weight eventually regain more weight than they lost.

So what are we going to do about it?

- **Stop dieting!** We know it doesn't work. We know it actually works against you.
- **Eat when you are hungry and stop when you are comfortable.** When we diet we force ourselves *not* to listen to our natural hunger cues. When we do this, we also tend *not* to listen to our "comfortable" cues. We react to deprivation and not listening to hunger by overeating at times. In order to stop overeating, we need to stop dieting and start listening to when our body truly is hungry and truly is comfortable. But, unfortunately, all of this may be a little trickier for people with type 2 diabetes. The biochemistry of the disease is thought to alter natural hunger regulation, so you may have to pay attention to hunger and eating until you are comfortable within the specific plan that you have worked out with your Certified Diabetes Educator to keep your blood sugars normal.
- **Beware of calories you are drinking.** Your body tends not to feel satisfied by liquid calories, and opting for healthier beverages is an easy way to trim excess calories.

- **Slow down; you're eating too fast.** It takes at least 20 minutes for your brain to get the message that your stomach is officially "comfortable" and that you should stop eating. If you eat slowly, the brain has a chance to catch up with the stomach and you are more likely not to overeat. Here are some tips to help slow you down during your meal:

  - Slow down your meal and chew slowly too.

  - Don't eat standing up; your brain and stomach are more likely to register that you are eating if you are relaxed and enjoying the meal.

  - Drink a 12-ounce glass of water before or while eating a meal.

- **Start exercising!** Exercising helps your body in so many ways. It is one of the fastest ways to increase your "calories out" side of the equation. (See Step #10 in Chapter 4 for information about how to exercise if you don't like to exercise.)

- **Start counting carbohydrates, fats, and fiber** as often as you can to gain tight control of your blood sugar. I know counting is a big pain, but you don't have to do it all the time for the rest of your life. You might start counting your carbohydrates, fat, and fiber every day until your blood sugar levels are under control. Then you can do "check in" counting when trying out a new meal or snack if your blood sugar levels are staying within normal limits.

Logging what you eat and when you exercise will also help you and your dietitian or Certified Diabetes Educator better understand what small changes might take place to encourage weight loss.

To diet or not to diet

When the holidays have finally passed, 'tis the season to get dieting. It's the American way. But when it comes to shopping for a diet, it's buyer beware, according to a report from the Federal Trade Commission, released September 17, 2002. The researchers found that 55 percent of the weight-loss advertisements made at least one false or unsubstantiated claim. Does this really surprise us? Nearly half the ads claimed you could lose weight without dieting and exercise.

All fad diets promoting fast and furious weight loss generally don't work over the long haul. Some of us have already figured this out on our own but we can't quite stop ourselves from perking up and asking "How'd you do it?" every time we hear someone say they lost 20 pounds. We can't quite tune out the countless TV commercials we see daily for weight-loss programs and products.

If you are going to partake of a fad diet in the new year, go in forewarned that with fad diets, weight loss is temporary. A USDA study found that pretty much any fad diet will help you take off the pounds, but there's not much evidence that they'll help you keep the weight off. Fad diets often work in the short run because they are low-calorie diets in disguise.

Weight loss fact: the only way to lose weight without medication or surgery is to consume less energy (calories) than your body needs. No magic ingredients or food combinations will change this basic metabolic fact.

But most people who successfully lose weight return to their old eating habits sooner or later and regain most of the lost weight within two years (Denke, M. "Metabolic effects of high-protein, low-carbohydrate diets" *Am J Cardiol* [2001]; 88:59–61). That's why the way of eating you choose needs to be practical and healthful for a lifetime. Most fad diets are neither of these things.

Nobody wants to hear this, but there is no miracle remedy or diet for losing weight. Your best bet is to stick with the proven method of eating less, eating healthier, and exercising more.

So, say you are ready to try to eat less, eat healthy, and exercise more. Which diet or way of eating is the best way to do that? The popular low-carbohydrate/high-protein way? The low-fat/higher-carbohydrate way? Or, the moderate-fat way (but emphasizing the better fat, carbohydrate, and protein choices)? Each will work in the short run as long as the calories you take in are less than the calories you are expending. But, healthwise, which is best?

Where are the fruits and vegetables?

Instead of "Where's the beef?" one crucial question to ask when looking at these different diets is "Where are the fruits and vegetables?"

Some studies have shown that the obesity levels are lowest among those who eat seven or more servings of fruits and vegetables a day (a key finding from research from the Produce for Better Health Foundation, Press Release October 21, 2002). And perhaps it isn't a coincidence that, as Americans have been getting fatter over the last 10 years, fruit and vegetable consumption has declined nearly 14 percent, nationwide, during the same period. We all know fruits and vegetables are good for us. Well, guess what? They are mostly carbohydrate (vegetables will have some plant protein too).

A cup of steamed broccoli contains 44 calories, 4.5 grams protein, 8 grams carbohydrate, 0.5 grams of fat, and 4.7 grams of fiber. And a large apple contains 125 calories, 0.4 grams protein, 32 grams carbohydrate, 0.7 grams of fat, and 4.2 grams fiber. Both are brimming with a good dose of healthful carbohydrate, complete with fiber.

? Are you losing fat, lean body mass, or water weight?

No one will argue that the main goal of weight loss is to lose body fat and not lean body mass (muscle). Water loss is fast and temporary, so eventually your body is going to need to restore the balance of water and will gain lost water pounds back.

The ideal weight loss diet should provide enough carbohydrate to prevent protein/muscle breakdown, enough good-quality protein to meet the normal needs of protein turnover, and enough fat to meet essential fatty acid requirements.

The following covers each of these three major diet groups, their strengths and their weaknesses, and some tips for you to keep in mind, should you decide (after consulting your doctor or dietitian) that's the program for you.

High protein/low carbohydrate. Atkins, South Beach, The Zone, Protein Power, Sugar Busters: do these diets sound familiar? These types of diets do encourage fast weight loss in the first week, though what's initially happening here is mostly water loss. The body needs a constant supply of glucose energy, so without a lot of carbohydrates in the diet, body glycogen stores (the way the body stores some extra carbohydrates) are used up. For each gram of glycogen lost, two to four grams of body water are lost as well. One study demonstrated that the greater weight loss on a low-carbohydrate/high-protein diet plan is accounted for by losses in body water (Denke, M. "Metabolic effects of high-protein, low-carbohydrate diets" *Am J Cardiol* 88 [2001]:59–61).

The American Heart Association has officially cautioned the public on high-protein diets. In an advisory to clinicians, it concluded that people who follow high-protein diets are at risk for "compromised vitamin and mineral intake, as well as potential cardiac, renal, bone, and liver abnormalities overall" (*Circulation* 104, no. 15 [2001]: 1869–74). According to this American Heart Association Science Advisory report, "the beneficial effects on blood lipids and insulin resistance are due to the weight loss, not the change in caloric composition." The advisory also reminds us that there are no long-term scientific studies to support the overall efficacy and safety of the various and sundry high-protein diets.

One *plus* with this type of diet is that you can lose weight fast, which can give some people the impetus they need to make longer-term changes in their eating habits and lifestyle. But losing weight too fast can be a problem, too. When weight loss is too fast, changes in body composition, especially the loss of lean body mass, can compound the problem of being overweight in the long run. When you lose weight quickly, you tend to lose some lean body mass (muscle protein), but when you gain the weight back quickly, it tends to come back as mostly body fat.

The other plus: there is some evidence that higher-protein diets are more satiating. People feel fuller and tend to eat less after a meal with a high-protein content (more than 25 percent of calories from protein). High-protein foods tend to move more slowly from the stomach to the intestine than high-carbohydrate (refined) foods, so your stomach tends to feel full longer.

According to one report, two of the five high-protein diets on the market score slightly better nutritionally than the others. The Zone and Sugar Busters diets at least do not severely restrict carbohydrate to fewer than 100 grams a day and total fat and saturated fat are not excessive (more than 30 percent of calories from fat and 10 percent of calories from saturated fat). (*Circulation* 104, no. 15 [2001]: 1869–74.)

The bottom line: this way of eating *can't* and *shouldn't* be continued over a long period of time. These diets are generally associated with higher intakes of fat, saturated fat, and cholesterol, if the protein choices come mostly from animal sources. In the long term, very-high-protein diets may increase the risk of atherosclerosis. One study showed that this diet increases serum cholesterol levels and may increase the risk of coronary heart disease by more than 50 percent with long-term use (*J Am Coll Nutr* 19 [2000]:578–590). Thomas Lee, MD, commented in the March 2002 issue of the "Harvard Heart Letter" that for most people eating a high-protein diet (including a lot of cheese, red meat, and other high-fat foods), their cholesterol levels, especially LDL (bad) cholesterol, go way up and that limiting foods that lower LDLs (such as high-fiber plant foods) only intensifies this problem.

Here's another fact that you need to keep in mind with high-protein diets: the more protein you eat, the more calcium you excrete. High-protein diets, when followed for a long time, can increase your risk of osteoporosis by increasing calcium excretion, and place an extra stress on the kidneys, which are removing high amounts of nitrogen waste products from the high protein intake, particularly during times of high water loss from perspiration or low fluid intake contributing to dehydration.

Short-term consequences of following a diet high in protein and fatty foods include dehydration, diarrhea, weakness, headaches, dizziness, and bad breath. This type of diet also tends not to include sufficient fruits and vegetables for overall good health.

Where does the South Beach Diet fit into this? Similar to the Atkins diet, the South Beach Diet is low in carbohydrates during its first phase. But in the second phase, the plan "legalizes" healthful carbohydrates such as whole grains, high-fiber cereal, and most fruit, and allows sparing amounts of chocolate, red wine, and previously banished foods, such as low-fat yogurt.

High carbohydrate/very low fat. The biggest positive to this type of diet is that it can lead to healthy eating as long as the diet recommends high fiber intakes and lower-glycemic-index carbohydrates (vegetables, beans, whole grains, and some fruits tend to have lower glycemic indexes), and provides sufficient essential fatty acids and fat-soluble vitamins from the fats that are eaten.

Another plus is that the diet quality tends to be better with this type of diet compared to the low-carbohydrate diets. A U.S. study of popular diets demonstrated that the diet quality (measured by dietary variety and intake of five food groups, and suggested amounts of fat, saturated fat, and sodium) is higher in high-carbohydrate diets and lowest in low-carbohydrate diets. The same study also detected another plus to high-carbohydrate eating: body mass index (BMI) is lower in people following high-carbohydrate diets and highest in people on low-carbohydrate diets (Kennedy et al., "Popular diets: correlation to health, nutrition, and obesity" *JADA* 101 [2001]:411–420).

The trouble with a high-carbohydrate/low-fat diet is that some might be tempted to fill up on higher-glycemic-index carbohydrates (refined starchy foods and concentrated sugar), which are rapidly digested and can cause a large increase in blood glucose and insulin after meals. Some clinical trials have reported less weight loss on high-glycemic-index diets compared to low-glycemic-index diets, and some short-term feeding studies found that as glycemic index goes down, satiety (a satisfied feeling of fullness) tends to go up (Pawlak et al., "Should obese patients be counseled to follow a low-glycemic-index diet?" *Obes Rev* 3, no. 4 [2002]: 235–43).

The bottom line: choose mostly smart carbohydrates (higher fiber, higher nutrient carbohydrates with lower glycemic indexes) and make sure you are getting enough protein and smart fat (extra virgin olive oil, canola oil, fish, avocado, nuts, and so on) to meet your body's needs.

A moderate, more balanced way of eating. This way of eating tends not to be studied as a diet, so there is very little research on this type of diet and weight loss. But if you combined the best part of the high-carbohydrate diet with the best part of the high-protein diet, would you have the best of both worlds? In other words, make your eating plan a little higher in protein and make sure your carbohydrate choices are smarter. In one study, a low-fat diet with 25 percent calories from protein was found to produce a significant reduced calorie intake and greater weight and fat loss over a six-month period compared to a low-fat diet with a lower protein intake—12 percent calories from protein (*Int J Obes Relat Metab Disord* 23 [1999]: 528–536). A realistic, higher protein, weight-reducing diet was associated with greater body fat loss and lower blood pressure compared to a high carbohydrate/high fiber diet in high-risk overweight and obese women, according to a more recent study (*Nutrition Journal* 10 [2011]: 40).

My money is on the best of both "diet" worlds, so to speak. By emphasizing the higher fiber, nutrient-rich carbohydrate foods (whole grains, beans, fruits, and vegetables) and the lower-fat protein sources (lean meats, fish, skinless poultry, low-fat dairy, and/or vegetable protein sources such as beans, whole grains, nuts, and seeds) and including smart fats.

Look for the following in a weight-loss plan:

- Does it consider your current habits, preferences, and risk factors?
- Does it set realistic weight loss goals (one to two pounds per week)?
- Does it have a daily intake of *at least 45 percent calories from carbohydrate?* For a woman eating at least 1,200 calories, this would compute to at least 135 grams of carbohydrate a day, and 169 grams for a man eating at least 1500 calories.
- Does it have a carbohydrate intake of *at least* 150 grams per day?
- Does it include all of the food groups?
- Does it emphasize fiber?
- Does it recommend regular exercise?
- Is it based on changing life-long eating habits?

2. I have couch potato-itis

If the first thing doctors told you to do after being diagnosed with type 2 diabetes was "lose weight," then the second thing they probably told you was to "start exercising." The bottom line is that physical activity can make the difference between losing weight and not losing weight, blood sugar control and out-of-control blood sugar, going on insulin and not having to go on insulin, taking a high dose of insulin and taking a lower dose of insulin. Regular exercise has been shown to lower triglyceride levels in the blood and lower blood pressure after only 10 weeks. The risk of heart attack and cancer also decreases with regular exercise.

Exercise does much more than reduce risk factors; it has psychological benefits too. It just plain makes you feel better. It tends to encourage better sleep, and it gives you more energy throughout the day. It helps you feel better about your body, even if pounds haven't been lost, and it helps reduce depression and stress.

I can go over and over all the various and sundry benefits (immediate and down the road) of exercise and physical activity, and I can even hold your hand and follow you around for a month, to help you get in the habit of exercising. But sooner or later it is all going to come back to one person: you. Ultimately, you have to take responsibility for yourself.

The first step, other than accepting that you have diabetes, is to commit to trying exercise for one month, remembering to start slowly. To see major benefits in your blood sugar control, exercising five to six times a week (even if it is just for

15 minutes each time) is helpful. At the end of one month you should hopefully have experienced many of the psychological and physiological benefits to exercise and you will be, let's hope, adequately "hooked." So let's look at how to get started:

- Visit your doctor and make sure you can proceed with your plans to start exercising.

- Don't make it a big weight loss contest—focus on health and gaining better control of your blood sugar.

- It has to be fun or you are definitely not going to stick with it.

- Find out what your exercise preferences/needs are and try to consider them when making your exercise plans.

- Do you like exercising outdoors or indoors?

- Do you like to exercise alone, with a partner, or with a group?

- Do you like the gym atmosphere?

- What time of day would you be most likely to stick to exercising?

- Do you have any physical limitations that need to be considered? If you have joint limitations, for example, water aerobics or swimming can be a great starting place.

- What do you like to do? Even if your answer is watching television or talking, they can be worked into your exercise program. If you like to talk, walking with a partner might be the ticket. It you like to watch television, then home exercise equipment that you can do in the comfort of your family room or bedroom might be your most practical option.

Every little bit helps

Even if you can't imagine exercising 30 minutes or more in one sitting, split it up into three 10-minute mini-workouts. Ten minutes of activity here and there does add up to health benefits for your body. Any way that you can increase your activity throughout your day will help your cause.

Here are some tips to keep you exercising month after month:

- Wherever you choose to exercise (gym, park, or pool) it should be **no more than 20 minutes away** from your home or work.

- **Start an exercise journal** or incorporate the information into your "A Day at a Glance Journal" in Chapter 4. You will be able to see progress. You will also be able to trace back situations when the exercise helped lower your blood sugar.

- **Have a plan B.** Have some indoor options for exercise planned. During the winter, it might be too cold to exercise outdoors, or it might get dark earlier and you are concerned about safety. Or perhaps you get stuck in traffic and don't get home in time to make your exercise class. Your plan B could be riding your stationary bike or playing one of your exercise videos.

- **Plan variety into your exercise schedule.** If you go to a dance class two times a week, you might want to add a walking workout a couple of times a week. I have three different types of exercise I do in any week (what can I say? I get bored easily). I go to a cardio hip-hop class two to three times a week and fill in the rest of my week with walks around the neighborhood and evening rides on my stationary bike (while I watch my favorite nighttime television shows).

- **Make different types of activity part of your normal day.** These may include walking the dog, taking a flight of stairs, or walking during part of your lunch break.

- **Check in with a personal trainer every three months.** They can give you specific things you can do, given your personal experiences and preferences. A "check in" session will run you about $30 to $100. Can call the American College of Sports Medicine for a list of personal trainers in your area (*www.acsm.org*).

To keep yourself from getting bored, don't be afraid to **try something new**. You could sign up for a class with your local parks and recreation program or through a community college. You could try a session of country western dance class, and then try yoga, water aerobics, tai chi, or tap the next session.

You've got to **choose exercise that you actually enjoy**. Of course, it is a matter of personal preference, but a large majority of people enjoy walking the most. It's easy, free, and only requires a pair of comfortable shoes. Look around your home or work for lakes or parks that you can walk around after dinner, during the lunch hour, or on the weekends.

If you are the type of person who is inspired by reaching a goal each day, consider wearing a pedometer! Throughout the day you will see the numbers on your pedometer increase, and if you have a certain number of steps to reach each day, this will really motivate you to keep moving and walking! Talk to your doctor, but 10,000 steps is the number where many very active people end up at the end of the day after really trying hard to get those steps in. Your doctor might encourage you to start with 5,000 steps and work your way up to 10,000.

Home exercise equipment

Stationary and recumbent (in which your back is supported) bicycles are very successful with former couch potatoes. You can literally go from the couch to the bicycle. Position a fan in front of the bicycle if you like. There are a few things to consider when picking out an exercise bike:

- Make sure the seat is adjusted to your body correctly.

- Make sure the seat is wide and comfortable.

- If you opt for a stationary bike, consider the type where the fly wheel gives you a breeze (helping you to cool off) and the handles move (because this prevents leaning).

- Many people make the mistake of buying inexpensive exercise equipment. I know this is tempting. Well-made equipment, the kind that will last a lifetime, will run you around $800 (give or take a couple of hundred). This is shocking, I know. But if you buy the cheaper stuff that creaks when you use it, it will inevitably break or you will tire of it quickly because it isn't as comfortable to use. Isn't buying one of the well-made pieces of equipment better than buying three cheaper pieces that you will stop using after a few months? Many stores offer payment plans in which the cost is about $20 or $30 a month. There are also places that sell used exercise equipment, which can shave quite a bit off the price.

Another home exercise no-no: don't buy exercise equipment through catalogs or television commercials. You want to try it out before you buy it. Put your sweats on and go to the sports equipment store. Tell them you want to try it out for 20 or 30 minutes. Only then will you be able to tell whether you can comfortably exercise on it for at least 30 minutes at home.

If you want to research the better designed pieces of exercise equipment, look up *Consumer Reports* online or at your local library—they rate exercise equipment every year. But remember, the only way to know for sure if you like it is to just get on and try it.

3. The junk food junkie

Are you a junk food junkie? For food to qualify as "junk food" it usually contributes a high number of calories for a low nutritional value.

The problem with these types of foods (a high number of calories within a small food volume, low fiber and water content, and low nutrients) is that they tend to cause a decrease in satiety (fullness and satisfaction when eating), which can encourage people to over-consume calories, potentially leading to obesity. Does that sound familiar, America?

A big portion of what I would call "junk food" essentially falls into the categories of "snack food" and "fast food." Popular snack foods are usually either packaged or commercially prepared such as chips, cheese puffs, candy bars, snack cakes, and cookies. The contribution of snack-type food to our total calorie consumption should not be underestimated. Between 1977 and 1996, the contribution of snack calories to total calories for American children between 2 and 5 years of age increased by 30 percent, according to an article in the Chilean medical journal, *Revista Medica de Chile*. Junk food is also quickly purchased at fast-food chains across the country in the form of french fries, chicken nuggets, shakes, soda, and so on, and we all know how pervasive fast food is in our current American culture. Then there are certain food categories such as breakfast cereals that seem innocent enough but include various products that could definitely be considered junk food, as they mostly contain sugar or high fructose corn syrup and white flour or milled corn.

Keep in mind that what is or is not considered junk food can depend on who you ask. Some might say pizza is junk food, for example, whereas I personally don't consider it 100-percent junk food, because it contributes nutrients through real foods such as cheese and tomato sauce. Add whole-wheat or part whole-wheat pizza crust and some veggies as toppings and pizza completely exits the junk food category. You just can't compare the nutrients in pizza to the nutrients (or lack there of) in a can of soda or a bag of chips.

Real food versus junk food

As if consuming the "junk" in junk food weren't bad enough, one of the worst detriments to eating junk food is that it tends to replace real food—food that contributes necessary and beneficial nutrients. Got milk? When people drink a lot of soda, for example, they are usually not getting plenty of low-fat dairy in their diet, along with other healthful beverages such as unsweetened green tea or pulpy orange juice blended with carrot juice. When they are snacking on chips and cookies, they are usually not loading up on fruits and vegetables.

Taking the "junk" out of junk food

No matter where you are, opt for food and beverage choices that are comprised mostly of whole foods or ingredients that offer nutrients along with calories. Enjoy freshly squeezed orange juice or a whole-wheat bagel instead of soda or donuts. Buy a bean burrito, pizza topped with vegetables, or a grilled chicken sandwich on a whole grain bun instead of tortilla chips with processed cheese sauce, frozen pizza rolls, or fried chicken pieces and french fries. Choose a 100-percent whole-wheat cracker made with canola oil, for example, or make a cheese and fruit plate to snack on instead of a bowl of cheese puffs.

No matter what we do, typical fast food seems to make us eat more

Eating large amounts of food at a rapid rate is defined as "gorging" and this is *not* a healthy way to eat, in part because we are more likely to take in an excessive amount of calories. You want to eat in a slow and mindful way so that you enjoy your food and your brain is aware of the eating process and is given time to tell your stomach when it is comfortable and satisfied. No good can come from eating large amounts of food quickly, and this is exactly what people tend to do when they eat fast food.

But is it the actual fast food that causes us to eat more than is needed or is it how much we are given and how we tend to eat fast food that seems to encourage gorging? A study from the Children's Hospital in Boston used teens from 13 to 17 years of age and exposed them to three types of fast food meals (all including chicken nuggets, french fries, and cola). In one meal, they were served a lot of fast food at one time. In another, a lot of fast food was served in smaller portions, but almost at the same time. And in the third test meal, a lot of fast food was served in smaller portions over 15-minute intervals. The researchers analyzed how many calories were consumed by the teens in these three situations.

What they found was it didn't seem to matter how the large amount of fast food was served—the teens still ate about half of their daily calorie needs in that one meal. The researchers suggested that certain factors inherent to fast food might be promoting excessive calorie intake:

- Low in fiber.
- High in palatability (pleasant tasting).
- High in calorie density (a high number of calories for a small volume).
- High in fat content.
- High in sugar in liquid form.

My suggestion is to choose fast-food options high in fiber (it exists!) that have a lower calorie density and a lower fat content, and to completely avoid sugar in liquid form when eating fast food. This means choosing fast-food restaurants that have these types of offerings.

? Do commercials for junk food make you eat more?

Let's start off by agreeing that the majority of food commercials targeting children are for junk foods—foods high in fat, sugar, or salt and low in nutritional value. And if you've ever wondered if watching advertisements for assorted types of processed food products encourages children to eat more, some research suggests your suspicions are more than warranted.

Researchers from the University of Liverpool in the United Kingdom exposed 60 children, between the ages of 9 and 11, of varying weights, to both food advertisements and toy advertisements, followed by a cartoon and free food.

More food was eaten after the food advertisements than after the commercials for toys. Interestingly, the obese children increased their consumption of food the most (134 percent) compared to overweight children (101 percent) and normal weight children (84 percent).

I'm not surprised by these results. The whole point of food advertising is to encourage consumption of the product. If it didn't work, why would food and beverage companies continue to spend millions on advertising? It does appear, though, that obese and overweight children are particularly vulnerable to this, and that in itself is alarming and worth noting to appropriate government agencies.

We can take junk food advertising out of our lives by limiting television viewing. Certain shows seem to attract more junk food commercials than others, so take note, parents, and discourage the viewing of these shows whenever possible. There are high-tech alternatives out there as well that help eliminate exposure to commercials, such as TIVO (which you can use to fast forward through commercials) or the use of DVDs.

Basically, to take the junk out of junk food, we need to choose foods and products with whole or real foods as often as possible and that contain fewer certain ingredients such as sugar, high-fructose corn syrup, milled grains, and partially hydrogenated oil.

Chapter 3

Everything You Ever Wanted to Ask Your Dietician

Diet and type 2 diabetes

You have questions about your diet and diabetes, and, hopefully, I have answers for you. This chapter isn't meant to substitute for consulting with a dietitian or Certified Diabetes Educator (CDE) and working with him or her to fine tune your diet and lifestyle to normalize your blood sugar. It's designed to be a helpful complement to working with him/her. If, after reading this chapter, you still have questions on food, diet, and diabetes, write them down as they pop into your mind and bring that list with you the next time you see your dietitian or CDE.

? Do you have a list of foods I cannot eat?

No—there isn't a list of foods you absolutely cannot eat. All foods, albeit in smaller serving sizes, can be worked into a particular eating plan. If dietitians tell you that you can't have something anymore, it will only make you feel deprived and angry, and you will only want to have that food more. You ultimately decide what to eat. And it is you who will learn to associate certain foods, in certain amounts and in certain combinations, with higher blood sugar.

❓ How can I enjoy the holiday season with type 2 diabetes?

You can have your pumpkin pie and eat it too during the holiday season, even if you have type 2 diabetes. Finding out you are at risk for developing diabetes is not the time to give up or run scared; it's time to make some simple switches in your diet and lifestyle. These changes will help you feel better too!

With the following tips you can get closer to your goal of feeling great and getting your diabetes under good control, all while eating the foods you love.

1. **With diabetes it's not only what you eat but also how much that impacts blood sugar levels.** Encourage sensible serving sizes by using small plates and bowls whenever possible and comparing your meat serving to a deck of cards or the palm of your hand (about three ounces cooked) and your side of rice or potatoes to a rounded ice-cream scoop (half a cup).

2. **When eating out, become a student of the menu.** Most fast-food and restaurant chains have nutrition information for their menu items available on their Websites or listed right on their menus. Take a look ahead of time and find menu items that appeal to you and contain roughly the amount of carbohydrates suggested by your dietitian or doctor for that meal. When available, also look for these options on the menu:

   • The petite serving of meat.

   • The cup of soup instead of a bowl.

   • A side serving or "half" serving of salad compared to the full size, especially if the soup or salad has carbohydrate-containing grains or beans. If the dressing is sweet, like Catalina or raspberry vinaigrette, order the dressing on the side and only add one tablespoon, which is about 3 to 5 grams of carbohydrates.

   • If ordering a pasta entrée or a sandwich, choose the whole grain option if possible.

3. **Eat your meal slowly, savoring every bite by letting your taste buds truly taste all the flavors and textures**. It takes at least 20 minutes for your brain to get the message that your stomach is officially "comfortable" and that you should stop eating, so slow down to avoid overeating. You may find you're more likely to be satisfied with half of what was served, and then you can take the rest home for a super enjoyable lunch the next day.

4. **Enjoy low- or zero-calorie beverages throughout the holiday season.** There are so many options to choose from now; in fact, recent data from the CDC show that during a 10-year period, the percentage of people selecting diet beverages has increased to about one-fifth of the U.S. population. Some of my favorites include unsweetened tea, mineral or seltzer water, and diet cola. Make them festive by ordering them with a wedge of lemon or lime.

5. **Maximize the foods that help keep your levels steady.** Whole foods such as whole grains, buckwheat and oats, beans and soybeans, and ground flaxseed can help improve blood sugar control and help keep insulin levels steady. You also can balance any carbohydrate-containing foods in your meal with options such as lean meats, poultry, fish, avocados, salad, vegetables, eggs, and cheese.

6. **Holiday desserts are non-negotiable!** Most of us look forward to enjoying certain favorite holiday treats when November and December roll around. The good news is that you can have your pumpkin pie and eat it too by doing three things: serve yourself petite portions of the desserts you love, enjoy them mindfully by being in the moment and truly tasting every bite, and count the carbohydrates contributed by the dessert into your meal carbohydrate budget.

7. **Employ your arsenal of delicious and diabetes-friendly potluck dishes** when going to holiday get-togethers. Bring something you are really looking forward to, and others will likely enjoy your lighter dish as well. I have an assortment of these recipes on my Website, *www.recipedoctor.com*, including Easy Pumpkin Pie, Potato Casserole, Citrus Salmon Salad, Zucchini Casserole, Wheat Cloverleaf Rolls, Garlic and Herb Twice-Baked Potatoes, and Best Bread Pudding.

8. **Now is a great time to crank your activity level up a notch!** Staying active and exercising regularly reduces your risk of type 2 diabetes and helps those with diabetes improve their blood sugar and insulin levels. It also helps keep your metabolism all fired up at a time when you are likely to be eating and drinking a little extra. Regular exercise can help improve your mood and promote more positive feelings about your body. Most of us are more likely to stay active over the holidays if we find activities that we truly enjoy and do with a friend.

One last tip: measuring your blood sugar levels about one and a half to 2 hours after eating, if you have diabetes, will tell you whether your blood sugar is within normal limits, high, or low. This becomes especially important during the holidays, when you might be eating and exercising a little differently.

Are there any food tricks I need to know to help prevent/treat type 2 diabetes?

Studies support the importance of including whole grains, fruits, vegetables, and low-fat dairy in the diet of people with diabetes. An emphasis should be on balancing carbohydrates with protein and smart fats (monounsaturated fats and omega-3 fats) when possible. Remember, the following foods, when eaten alone, even in large amounts, are not likely to cause a significant rise in blood sugar because they contain few carbohydrates:

- Meat.
- Poultry.
- Fish.
- Avocados.
- Dark green veggies and salad vegetables.
- Eggs.
- Cheese.
- Mushrooms (crimini mushrooms, for example, contain about 3 grams of carbs in one cup).

Here are some specific food suggestions that may help as well:

- **Fiber:** The chronic consumption of low amounts of fiber has been associated with an increased risk of type 2 diabetes as well as cancer, obesity, and heart disease.
- **Omega-3 fatty acids:** These may be especially helpful for people with type 2 diabetes who are at increased risk of heart disease.
- **Soy**: Soy may help people with diabetes control their blood sugar. Soy has been shown to make cells more responsive to insulin.
- **Buckwheat:** New research shows that extract of buckwheat lowered meal-related blood sugar levels by 12–19 percent when given to rats. Buckwheat does appear to be a potentially "magical" intact whole grain for people with diabetes. So how do you get more buckwheat into your diet? Look for buckwheat soba noodles in your supermarket, and start cooking with buckwheat groats. (They can be cooked similar, to other intact whole grains.) And check out new recipes using buckwheat groats and buckwheat soba noodles in the recipe chapter.

- **Green tea:** I'm a big green/white tea advocate because of all the antioxidant plant compounds (polyphenols) it provides, but there are possibly bigger benefits for people with pre- or type 2 diabetes. More investigation needs to be done, but a review of 17 randomized clinical trials suggests green tea consumption was associated with lower fasting blood sugar levels and lower fasting insulin levels. Lower blood levels of hemoglobin A1c (a marker of long-term presence of excess glucose in the blood) were also noted. These promising benefits appeared to be more pronounced in people with metabolic syndrome risk factors. Black tea doesn't have as many of the polyphenol plant compounds as green tea.

- **Whey protein:** Whey protein hydrolysates may prove to be helpful antidiabetic agents, according to new research with obese diabetic mice. The whey protein improved blood glucose clearance, reduced elevated insulin levels, and remarkably restored the ability of pancreas cells to release insulin in response to glucose. Past research has linked consumption of low fat dairy with a reduction in risk of type 2 diabetes and specific amino acids in milk have been reported to stimulate insulin secretion.

- **Cinnamon:** Several studies have been done suggesting cinnamon has a possible blood sugar lowering effect. The results of one study of 60 people suggest that less than half teaspoon of ground cinnamon a day reduces blood sugar in people with type 2 diabetes (*Diabetes Care* 26 [2003]: 3215–8). Results from another study suggest six grams of cinnamon (about two teaspoons) added to a hot cereal containing 50 grams of carbohydrate may help lower blood glucose levels after meals in normal weight and obese adults (*J Acad Nutr Diet* [November 2012]: 112(11): 1806–9). More research needs to be done but in the meantime, especially if you like cinnamon, sprinkle some in your morning cereal (hot or cold), coffee or lattes, and add it to your yogurt or smoothies.

- **Cocoa:** Cocoa may help control diabetes, according to a mice study from Penn State University. Cocoa powder is low in fat and low in sugar but contributes a lot of polyphenolic plant compounds. In the study, the mice diet was supplemented with cocoa (the human equivalent of about 10 tablespoons) and plasma insulin levels, weight gain, and liver triglyceride levels were all lower than the mice without cocoa supplementation. Dark chocolate contains these polyphenols as well, but, depending on the source, can have added fat, sugar, and calories that may outweigh these benefits. More research needs to be done in humans of course, but in the meantime, you might consider adding unsweetened cocoa powder to hot and cold cereal, smoothies, yogurt, and milk. And, if you are going to enjoy some chocolate, consider dark chocolate over milk or white chocolate (which don't have any or very little polyphenols).

- **Ground flaxseed:** There is some research suggesting there are health benefits for people with diabetes. (More on flaxseed in Chapter 4.)

- **Walnuts:** Nuts are wonderful whole foods that provide a balance of smart fats with some protein and fiber and phytochemicals along with a small amount of carbohydrates. Walnuts are highest in plant omega-3s. So I wasn't surprised to see a study recently that found that 2 ounces of walnuts a day improved arterial wall function (endothelial) in overweight adults with extra body fat surrounding organs in the abdominal area. This means there could be some awesome heart disease risk reduction benefits for people with (or at risk for developing) type 2 diabetes. And by the way, multiple studies have found that adding nuts to your diet does not lead to weight gain.

- **A glass of wine:** With dinner, a glass may help lower fasting blood sugar in some people with diabetes, suggests an Israeli study. The participants with the higher hemoglobin A1c levels saw the biggest reductions in fasting blood sugar. Along with potential health benefits, wine also brings 100 calories to the table, so you may need to trade these calories with another carbohydrate-rich food at dinner. Because 100 calories are equal to about 25 grams of carbohydrate, higher doses of alcohol can be dangerous. Before starting any amount of alcohol consumption, you should talk with your doctor or dietitian (Shai, I. et al., "Glycemic Effects of Moderate Alcohol Intake Among Patients with Type 2 Diabetes." *Diabetes Care*, 30 [December 2007]: 3011–3016).

- **Nopal:** Also known as the prickly pear and a member of the cactus family, nopal may help lower blood glucose when it is cooked (not raw). Nopal may help decrease carbohydrate absorption, thanks to its high amount of fiber and pectin (soluble fiber). More research needs to be conducted, but the amount suggested as helpful when eaten with meals is at least 3.5 ounces of broiled nopal stems.

- **Mushrooms** may have anti-diabetic properties! Stay tuned as more human research trial results become available, but put mushrooms on your list of potential foods with anti-diabetic properties. So far, preliminary data from human trials appear to mirror the encouraging

results in diabetic animal research, which includes potential in helping to lower plasma glucose, blood pressure, total cholesterol, and
serum triglycerides. Polysaccharides (possibly both alpha- and beta-
glucans) are the plant compounds in mushrooms that are thought to
be responsible for these desirable effects. The mechanism needs to
be confirmed, but some researchers suspect they work directly with
insulin receptors on target tissues. There may even be possible benefits from particular mushroom extracts helping to prevent cataracts
in people with diabetes, according to preliminary animal and lab
studies.

? I have a sweet tooth. Can I still eat some of my favorite desserts?

No one wants to be told they can't have something—especially when
that something is sugar. It only makes you want it more. And there is no reason
why people with diabetes can't have sugar, as long as they keep a few things in
mind. Bread and several other starches actually have almost the same effect on
blood sugar, in some people, as refined sugar does. But if the sugar-containing
meal actually contains more carbohydrates than your meal plan suggests (worked
out with your Certified Diabetes Educator), your blood sugar levels will likely go up.

With sugary foods, the rule is moderation, according to the American Diabetes
Association. If you are managing your blood sugar well, then you may have some
sugar, but you have got to play by a few rules:

- **Pay attention to portion sizes of sugary foods.** Keep servings moderate, such as a half cup of ice cream or three Oreo cookies.

- **Try to enjoy your dessert or high-sugar treat as part of a meal.**
  You will be less likely to overeat the treat if you have it with a meal,
  and the dessert will be less likely to send your blood sugar soaring if
  it's paired with other foods.

- **Substitute the sugar-containing food** for another carbohydrate-containing food in your personal diabetes meal plan. Otherwise you will
  not only increase the carbohydrates you're taking in, but you'll also
  increase your calories.

- **Monitor your blood glucose routinely** so you'll be aware of any
  negative effects from the sugary food.

- **Taking a brisk walk after the meal** to help lower blood sugar and
  burn some calories can also be helpful.

The lesson here is, go ahead and eat cake, but make it is a modest slice and have it with your meal. One last bit of advice: make sure these foods are truly satisfying, so you'll be happy with the moderate amounts.

? How can I do this without counting and measuring foods?

I don't like counting and measuring either. It automatically makes me feel "different" (and not in a good way) and, frankly, it can take the fun out of eating. I would strongly suggest checking out the carb-counting tips in Chapter 4 (including the one-page easy carb-counter guide). When you count carbohydrate, fat, and fiber grams every now and then, you sort of "check in" with how you are eating. When you compare it to blood sugar, this can be a great tool for you and your dietitian or diabetes educator. But if you really can't bring yourself to do it, the only answer is to monitor, monitor, monitor (your blood sugar, that is). Monitor your blood sugar three to six times a day, study your normal diet and the resulting blood sugar, and soon you will know which foods or meals work best.

The foods that cause high blood sugar may just need to be eaten in smaller amounts each time, combined with other foods, or coordinated with a change in medication or exercise just when that specific food/meal is eaten.

? Should I become vegetarian?

A total vegetarian diet can be high in carbohydrates, making normal blood sugar harder to achieve for some. If you choose to eat this way for other reasons, make sure you plan meals carefully to keep carbohydrates in check. You will need to depend heavily on plant foods that are higher in fat and protein, such as nuts, soybeans, and tofu, and plant foods rich in soluble fiber to help buffer the carbohydrate-induced rise in blood glucose. What might appeal more to most people is not necessarily a vegetarian diet, but just to plain eat more plant foods.

? I've heard there is a type of fiber that is good for people with type 2 diabetes. What is it?

Soluble fiber (fiber that is soluble, or dissolves in water) seems to be a vital component of blood glucose control for many people. It is found in peas and beans, oats and oat bran, barley, and some fruits and vegetables. Soluble fiber leaves the stomach slowly, so it makes you feel satisfied longer. I notice the feeling when I have beans with lunch, such as a bean burrito. (This is unusual because I am usually starving several hours after lunch.) Soluble fiber, which forms a gel within the intestinal tract, slows carbohydrate absorption and reduces the rise in blood glucose and insulin following the meal. Soluble fiber also has some disease-prevention benefits. Find out more about this in Chapter 4.

? Are the very-high-protein, very-low-carbohydrate diets good for people with diabetes?

These diets aren't good for anyone, but they can be dangerous for people with type 2 diabetes. People with diabetes are already at high risk for kidney disease (diabetes increases the rate at which the kidneys age), and excessive food protein and high blood pressure put even more stress on the kidneys. And people with diabetes do not have an increased need for protein as compared to those without diabetes. Most high protein diets are just fad diets in disguise—they aren't based on scientific and medical truths. Just think about it: fruits, vegetables, and whole grains are some of the most nutritious foods on Earth, contributing vitamins, minerals, phytochemicals, and fiber. These foods are made up of mostly—what? Carbohydrates. And though it is true that insulin is normally released into the blood stream when carbohydrates are eaten (in people without diabetes), the carbohydrates are stored as fat only if the amount of calories being eaten is greater than the amount needed by the body. So, carbohydrates don't automatically turn to fat unless you are eating too much.

Okay, so people say they have lost weight on these diets. The only thing that really counts is whether they were able to keep it off (and in this respect, most people haven't been as lucky). People may lose weight on these diets not because they are low in carbohydrates, but because they tend to be low in calories. People do lose weight quickly, but it isn't fat they're losing right away; it's mostly body water. As you continue the diet, you will lose some fat pounds, but at the same time, you are losing muscle tissue.

When you eat too few carbohydrates, your body automatically starts to sacrifice its protein tissue (from major organs and muscles) for energy. And when you gain the weight back, it is likely to be body fat, not muscle tissue. Over time, losing weight and gaining it back a few times causes you to get fatter and fatter and lose more and more muscle tissue. The liver and kidneys also have to work harder processing protein into energy than they would with carbohydrates.

? Are starchy foods, such as pasta, potatoes, and bread, fattening?

All of these foods are high in carbohydrate calories. Carbohydrates are only fattening when we eat more calories than our body needs. But this is also the case with foods high in protein and fat (*especially* fat). By including fruits and vegetables with these starches, we are more likely to keep our portions of these delicious starches reasonable. For example, when you fix pasta, add in some broccoli or carrots. When you make a sandwich with bread, have it with an apple, a wedge of melon, or a small bowl of fruit salad. With bread, you also have the opportunity to increase your daily fiber total by choosing bread that contains either whole grains or added soluble fiber.

? Is fat in food good or bad? I know it's bad for some diseases, but I also know it helps me control my blood sugar.

Over the past 15 years, things have become much more complicated. Fat in food is feared; its mere presence has been known to provoke massive anxiety on people. But the latest studies are showing us that some fats actually have a protective effect on our bodies in terms of heart disease and some cancers. They are also showing that there may not be one "right" amount of fat for all people; some people may fare better with more or less fat than others. Researchers are probably going to battle this out in the years to come, but in the meantime, you're trying to get a better handle on your blood sugar, your weight, and your risk of heart disease.

I don't blame you for being confused. Most of us health professionals are trying to figure it all out too. Yes, having a moderate-fat diet (30 to 35 percent of calories from fat) seems to add up to better blood sugar levels for some people with type 2 diabetes, compared to a very low-fat diet (10 to 20 percent of calories from fat). The fat helps slow down digestion in general, and "paces" the introduction of glucose (from carbohydrates eaten) into the blood stream. For a variety of reasons, fat also helps some people feel more satisfied after a meal or snack.

The tricky part is knowing how much is enough for the diabetic benefits but not too much that it increases your risk of other chronic diseases and weight gain. I would try to stick around 30 to 35 percent calories from fat, and see what effect it has on your blood sugar, weight, and blood lipid levels. This way you could still have about 15 to 20 percent calories from protein, leaving around 45 to 55 percent calories from carbohydrates (hopefully, mostly from whole grains, beans, fruits, and vegetables).

As part of this moderate-fat eating plan you absolutely *must* turn to the more heart-protective fats—the omega-3 and monounsaturated fats—to make up most of the 35 percent. This means using canola oil and extra virgin olive oil in cooking, choosing products that contain liquid canola oil or extra virgin olive oil (non-hydrogenated), including ground flaxseed in your diet, enjoying a handful of nuts on a daily basis, adding avocadoes and olives often, and eating fish two to three times a week.

If you like eating out, these new rules could cramp your style. Most fast food establishments and restaurants do *not* use liquid canola and olive oil (except maybe Italian or Mediterranean restaurants). But hang in there; there are all sorts of eating out tips for you in Chapter 8.

(?) Do blood lipids improve after people switch to mono-unsaturated fats and omega-3 fatty acids?

Yes! Some people who achieve good blood sugar control on low fat/high carbohydrate diets unfortunately see their LDL ("bad") cholesterol and triglycerides increase. But after adding omega-3 fatty acids and monounsaturated fats to total about 30 percent of calories from fat (or a little more), many people are able to improve their blood lipids without an increase in HgA1c (a blood test that, in essence, measures the 90-day average of blood sugar).

(?) The more I incorporate beans, which help my blood sugar, into my diet, the more gas I get. Is there anything I can do?

The fiber and some hard-to-digest complex carbohydrates in beans and legumes end up in the large intestine. The bacteria in the intestine then work on breaking down these substances, often giving off gas as a by-product, making you feel bloated. There are a few things you can do to minimize the gaseous effects of beans. Keep your serving of beans to about half a cup, to start with, and eat beans with a balanced meal containing protein, fat, and carbohydrates. There are also a couple of over-the-counter products that claim to alleviate bean-related digestive distress, such as the products available at *www.beanogas.com* and *www.bean-zyme.com*.

(?) What are bad and good cholesterol?

A high level of LDL cholesterol in the blood increases the risk of fatty deposits forming in the arteries, increasing the risk of heart attack. That's how LDL has gotten its nickname as the "bad" cholesterol. Elevated levels of HDL-cholesterol, on the other hand, seem to have a protective effect against heart disease, which is why it is fondly referred to as "good" cholesterol. One study revealed that, even in the participants with optimal LDL cholesterol levels (below 70 mg/dL), those with the highest amount of HDL cholesterol levels were at less risk for major cardiovascular events compared to those with the lowest amount (*New England Journal of Medicine*, September 27, 2007).

What about total serum (blood) cholesterol levels? Many people think lowering *food* cholesterol is the most important step toward lowering *blood* cholesterol. Actually, eating less saturated fat has a stronger effect on lowering blood cholesterol levels. Some studies, though, have found that consuming higher levels of cholesterol increases the risk of heart disease, even if it doesn't increase blood cholesterol levels.

? Is there anything I can do to lower my blood lipid levels?

The complete answer to this question could fill an entire book or at least a chapter! But here's the short version.

Tips to lower high serum cholesterol

General suggestions include cutting back on fat (especially saturated fat and trans fats) and dietary cholesterol within reason, while eating more fruits, vegetables, and foods rich in soluble fiber (such as oats and beans). Here are some specific suggestions:

- Eating whole grains when possible and limiting simple sugars may be helpful.
- The Portfolio Plan, which includes soy protein, almonds, plant sterol–enriched margarines, and soluble fiber–rich foods (oats, barley, psyllium, and vegetables such as okra and eggplant), has shown cholesterol-lowering benefits. The eating plan was developed by University of Toronto, and research with the plan has tested the combination of four cholesterol-lowering foods. It can be found at *http://portfolioeatingplan.com*.
- Green tea's abundant antioxidants may also lower total cholesterol by increasing intestinal excretion of cholesterol and bile acids (through your stool).

Tips to lower LDL cholesterol

- According to the Portfolio Plan, reductions in bad cholesterol result from diets containing almonds and diets that are either low in saturated fat or high in viscous fibers (fiber that tends to be "sticky" in the intestinal tract), soy protein, or plant sterols.
- You can cut out a lot of saturated fat and trans fat from your diet by limiting full-fat dairy products, higher-fat meats, poultry skin, stick butter and margarine, commercially made cookies and crackers, and fast-food french fries.

- Eating a vegetarian diet that includes cholesterol-lowering foods (such as soy milk, soy burgers, oats, nuts, bean soup, fruits, and vegetables, which have all been individually found to lower cholesterol levels) may lower lipid levels as much as some medications. In one study, after one month, LDL levels fell by 29 percent, a drop similar to that seen with some statin drugs.

- Some studies have suggested that ground flaxseed, about four tablespoons a day, can lower LDL cholesterol from nine to 18 percent, and total blood cholesterol up to nine percent. More clinical studies need to be done on ground flaxseed to confirm these positive effects, but there are so many other health benefits to a daily ground flaxseed regimen, that this seems to be the icing on the heart-healthy cake! For more tips, tricks, and recipes with ground flaxseed, check out my book *The Flax Cookbook*.

Tips to lower triglycerides

- Limit saturated fat and trans fats and replace them with monounsaturated fats such as olive oil, canola oil, and most nuts.

- Cut back on refined carbohydrates such as sweets, soft drinks, and white bread.

- Limit alcoholic drinks to no more than one a day for women and two a day for men. People with diabetes should check with their doctor before consuming any amount of alcohol.

- Ground flaxseed may contribute to lowering triglyceride levels.

- Maintain a healthy weight and exercise regularly.

- People with diabetes who also have high triglycerides and high LDLs benefit from including more monounsaturated fats (olive oil, canola oil, and avocado) and slightly fewer carbohydrates.

- People with diabetes may benefit from eating fish twice a week. If you don't like fish, you might consider discussing fish oil capsules (one to three grams a day) with your doctor.

Tips to lower C-reactive protein

A high level of this protein can signal blood vessel inflammation and a greater likelihood of a rupture.

- Eat salmon, albacore tuna, sardines, walnuts, and ground flaxseed for omega-3 fatty acids.

- C-reactive protein was also lowered in two Portfolio studies in which people consistently consumed four key foods: soy protein, plant sterol-ester enriched margarine, almonds, and high soluble fiber foods.
- Maintain a healthy weight and exercise regularly.

Food and blood sugar levels

? How and why do certain foods raise blood sugar more than others do?

The foods we eat contain different amounts and combinations of carbohydrates, protein, and/or fat. Vegetable oils contain all fat and granulated sugar contains all carbohydrate. Other foods contain two or three of these. All of the grams of the digestible carbohydrates we eat convert to glucose, whereas about half of the protein and 10 percent of the fat grams we eat converts to glucose after digestion.

Carbohydrates, protein, and fat show their peak effect on blood glucose at different times after a meal, too:

- **Simple sugars:** Peak 15 to 30 minutes after the meal.
- **Complex carbohydrates:** Peak one to one and a half hours after the meal.
- **Protein:** Peaks three to four hours after the meal.
- **Fat:** Peaks three hours after the meal.

How a particular food affects your blood glucose has to do, in part, with the combination of carbohydrate, protein, and fat in the food and the portion size you eat. How quickly the food is absorbed (and how quickly it affects blood glucose levels) also depends on factors such as the physical form of the food, whether the food is cooked, and what blood glucose levels were before the meal. One trick all people with diabetes have up their sleeves is dietary fiber. Dietary fiber, which is not digested by the body, causes other carbohydrates in the meal to be digested and absorbed more slowly, encouraging lower after meal blood sugar.

However, people respond differently to carbohydrates. The same meal eaten by different people might have varying effects on blood glucose levels. In some people, insulin becomes less effective after they eat high-animal-fat meals. This can also bring on high blood sugar. The only way to know for sure how your blood sugar responds to a particular meal is to test it before and two hours after the meal.

? What are the meals and foods that encourage higher blood sugar than would normally be expected?

Some health professionals call this the "pizza effect," so you can guess what is at the top of this list—pizza.

- **Pizza can result in surprisingly high post-meal blood sugar.** Suggestion: When people eat pizza, they usually just eat pizza and nothing else. So, right away we can change our post-meal blood sugar by *not* eating pizza alone. We will end up eating fewer slices of pizza too, if we pair one or two slices with a nice dark green salad, for example, with ample beans and raw veggies dressed with a dressing made with canola oil or extra-virgin olive oil. For additional tips on eating pizza a healthier way, check out Chapter 7.

- **Chinese food in general and chow mein and rice in particular.** Suggestion: use your carb-counting guide when you eat Chinese food. Keep chow mein or rice amounts within your carb budget and enjoy them with vegetables and fish or lean meat dishes.

- **Ramen noodles.** Suggestion: check the label to know how much of the dish you can have on your carb budget and enjoy it with other foods that won't increase your blood sugar, such as dark leafy greens, fish, lean meat, and so on. Note: Most Ramen packages list two servings per package so if you eat the whole 3 oz. package, double the amount of carbs, fat, and fiber listed on the label.

- **Bagels eaten plain (even one bagel can cause a problem for some).** Suggestion: start with half a bagel and eat it with some natural style peanut butter, cheese, or light cream cheese with lox.

- **Fried foods, such as fried chicken and french fries.** Suggestion: Enjoy fried foods in small amounts and pair them with other dishes that don't tend to raise blood sugar. Eat them slowly and pay attention to flavor and texture so the smaller amount will be satisfying.

- **Granola cereal.** Suggestion: start with a quarter of a cup served with plain Greek yogurt and see how that affects your blood sugar. Also, check the label and choose a granola that fits into your carb budget—one with less added sugar and more nuts and seeds, perhaps.

- **Pasta.** Suggestion: start the meal with a green salad or broth-based soup to bring the hunger down. Then try a one-cup serving of cooked whole grain pasta and/or gluten-free pasta made from quinoa or brown rice and see how it affects your blood sugar. Include the grams of carbs in your carb counting and enjoy the pasta with foods that don't tend to raise blood sugar such as fish, lean meats, vegetables, and so on.

- **High animal protein/fat meals, including those with lots of cheese, such as a big cheese omelet served with sausage or bacon, or a big steak dinner served with french fries.** Suggestion: when going for a high saturated fat meal, try to order or cook a smaller portion and add a lot of vegetables to the entrée (such as an omelet with lots of green vegetables, tomato, and avocado) while minimizing the cheese and processed meat accompaniments. Enjoy two strips or links instead of four. As far as french fries go, if you eat them slowly and really pay attention to taste and texture, you might be satisfied with about four bites of french fries instead of the whole pile.

- **Cold breakfast cereals.** Suggestion: choose whole-grain breakfast cereals (hot or cold) and add nuts and ground flaxseed to them to pump up the protein, fiber, and plant compounds. Add milk (low-fat milk, soy or almond) or fresh or frozen fruit to your cereal too as long as you figure the carbohydrate grams into your meal budget.

- **Baked potatoes.** Suggestion: count the grams of carbohydrate into your meal total and eat the skin (that's where a lot of the fiber and nutrients are) and top your potato with foods that add fiber and protein, such as beans, lean meat, dark green vegetables, Greek yogurt, and so on.

- **Watermelon and other melons.** Suggestion: count the carbs in your melon and stick to that serving size by serving yourself a small bowl of just that amount. If you start eating from the serving bowl, for example, you may over-consume because eating fresh watermelon is so easy to do.

(?) Are there foods that help prevent high blood sugar when they are paired with foods that tend to cause high blood sugar?

Adding plant foods that contribute some fat and/or protein to the meal (nuts, soy foods, olive and canola oil, flaxseed, avocado) seems to help minimize high blood sugar from notorious high-carbohydrate meals. But if you have a meal high in animal fat that usually brings on high blood sugar (pizza, high-fat breakfasts, and so on.), loading up on fiber (soluble fiber in particular) about 10 minutes before you start the meal may help. Higher soluble fiber plant foods will also help minimize high blood sugar from high-carbohydrate meals. As an appetizer, before you eat the entrée, try:

- A green salad with kidney beans and raw vegetables.
- A cup of vegetable or bean soup.
- A small serving of oat bran or oatmeal (before a problematic breakfast).
- Other high soluble fiber vegetables (see Chapter 4).
- Other high soluble fiber grain foods (see Chapter 4).
- Psyllium seed foods and supplements. (Powders without intestinal stimulants are available. Pysllium is also added to a couple of breakfast cereals.)

? Why do I have higher blood sugar after high-fat meals instead of high-carbohydrate meals?

Some people seem to have high blood sugar after meals particularly high in animal fats, such as bacon and eggs, or pizza topped with sausage and pepperoni. Some researchers think that in some people (particularly certain ethnicities such as Asians, Pacific Islanders, and African Americans), insulin becomes less effective after meals laden in animal fat. If you notice this happens with you, try having smaller portions of the fatty foods and add in some plant foods (fruits, vegetables, and whole grains, especially those rich in soluble fiber) and see if it makes a difference. Instead of bacon and eggs and hash browns, try one sausage link or bacon strip, one egg, and a buckwheat pancake or a bowl of oatmeal with fruit and nuts. Trade in your four slices of "meat lover's" pizza for two slices of "vegetable lover's" pizza plus a green salad with kidney beans and an olive oil vinaigrette, or a nice cup of vegetable or bean soup.

? What is the optimal percentage of carbohydrates, fat, and protein that helps control blood sugar?

According to Certified Diabetes Educators who I spoke with, about one-third of the people with type 2 diabetes tend to do better with an eating plan with 35 to 40 percent calories from fat (using mostly monounsaturated fats), whereas two-thirds tend to fair best with a 25 to 30 percent calories from fat. But there are many other food factors, other than the percentage of fat or carbohydrates, that can influence blood sugar control, such as total fiber/soluble fiber and whether proteins and fats come mostly from vegetable sources.

? What is your best breakfast if your blood sugar levels tend to be high in the morning?

This is so important for people with diabetes that we devoted an entire chapter to it! Check out the breakfast section in Chapter 8.

? What about wine? Does one glass at dinner help lower blood sugar?

A glass of red wine with dinner does seem to encourage lower blood sugar levels for some people, but it is very individual. For others, the opposite can happen—blood sugar levels seem to rise later that night. Sweeter wines tend to bring on higher blood sugar, so people tend to do better with red wines and drier wines. If you do have a glass of wine with dinner, check your blood sugar before bed, and, if you can, try testing your blood sugar at 2 or 3 a.m. every now and then. Let your Certified Diabetes Educator know if it seems to help normalize your blood sugar or elevate it. If sensitivity to alcohol or alcoholism is an issue, continue to avoid alcohol altogether.

? What alternative sweeteners should I buy if I want sweeteners without adding carbohydrates?

No- and low-calorie sweeteners come in handy if you are trying to reduce your calories from sugar, if you have diabetes and are trying to maintain normal blood sugar, and if you happen to like the taste of diet soda because regular soda tastes too sweet to you.

Can they really help with weight loss? According to a study by Dutch researchers, alternative sweeteners may have a pivotal role in our weight-loss and weight-maintenance plans. After reviewing many studies, they noted that the use of aspartame was associated with improved weight maintenance after a year. When no- and low-calorie sweetened beverages were substituted for regular, sweetened beverages (and calories were not restricted), people ended up eating fewer calories and weighing less, according to the results of two short-term studies (*American Journal of Clinical Nutrition*, February 1997).

Another Harvard Medical School study reported similar results in 1997. They assigned obese women to either consume or eliminate aspartame-sweetened foods for 16 weeks of a weight-reduction program. What happened? The women who were consuming aspartame lost significantly more weight overall and regained significantly less weight during the maintenance and follow-up phase (*American Journal of Clinical Nutrition*, February 1997).

I still wouldn't go hog wild for these no-calorie sweeteners, though, or consume unlimited amounts. I think moderation might be in order here too. Although not scientifically proven yet, some experts suspect that alternatively sweetened food and drink may psych out our bodies, so to speak, by telling our brains that something sweet is coming (as our taste buds sense the sweetness as we chew and swallow) and yet the body isn't getting the sugar calories it's expecting. This might, in some people, make them crave some real carbohydrate as a response to the unrequited consumption of simple carbohydrate. If there truly is this effect, I suspect this is less of an issue with moderate amounts of no- and low-calories sweeteners (one to two beverages a day) as compared to drinking no- and low-calorie sweetened beverages all day long.

? Which no- or low-calorie sweetener is right for me?

With so many no- and low-calorie sweeteners out there these days, how do you know which one to buy? Here's how they differ, and the pros and cons of each type.

Sucralose (Splenda)

Splenda contains the alternative sweetener sucralose, along with maltodextrin, which adds bulk so Splenda can be substituted cup-for-cup for sugar in recipes. Sucralose is 600 times sweeter than sugar. To make sucralose, they take a cane sugar molecule and substitute three hydrogen-oxygen groups with three chlorine atoms. After experimenting with Splenda in baking recipes, I have found the results are usually successful when I use half sugar and half Splenda. I still prefer to use less of the real thing, sugar, in baking though.

Pros:
- Sucralose has no calories. A small recent study raises the question of whether sucralose may raise blood sugar and insulin levels in some people in certain situations, but more research needs to be done to clarify this.
- You can bake with Splenda. Heat doesn't affect the sweetness.
- When it comes to baking and cooking, Splenda appears to be the best sweetener for the job.
- Of all the no- and low-calorie sweeteners that have been around a while, Splenda seems to have caused the least controversy from watchdog or consumer groups.

- After more than 110 studies (including animal and human studies), the FDA concluded that sucralose was shown to have no toxic or carcinogenic effects, no DNA altering, and does not pose reproductive or neurological risks to humans.

Cons:
- The bulking agents used in Splenda can add around 12 calories per tablespoon of the mixture (although the package does not list these calories).
- Splenda can change the texture in baking recipes and can add an "artificial" taste when used as the only sweetener in the recipe.

Saccharin (Sweet'N Low)

Saccharin, which is 300 times sweeter than sugar, is an organic molecule made from petroleum. After bladder cancer was found in male lab rats that were fed huge amounts of saccharin, the FDA proposed a ban on saccharin in 1977. But no ban was enacted, and the warning label on saccharin was dropped in 2000.

Pros:
- Heat doesn't affect its sweetness but can change its texture.

Cons:
- Since 1981, government reports have listed saccharin as an "anticipated human carcinogen." Although studies of heavy saccharin users don't support any link with cancer, certain subgroups, such as male heavy smokers, may be at increased risk. No human studies have shown evidence that saccharin causes cancer. It seems that the mechanism that causes saccharin to be a carcinogen to rats is not relevant to humans.

- The American Medical Association's Council on Scientific Affairs suggests that parents and caregivers limit young children's intake of saccharin, because little information is available on how it might affect them.

- Because saccharin can cross the placenta, the Council on Scientific Affairs suggests that women use saccharin carefully during pregnancy.

Aspartame (NutraSweet and Equal)

You would never guess that one of the most popular artificial sweeteners is actually a combination of two amino acids, phenylalanine and aspartic acid, which are then combined with methanol. It is 180–200 times sweeter than sugar.

About 70 percent of our aspartame intake is from soft drinks. The FDA has set the acceptable daily intake (ADI, the estimated amount a person can safely consume every day over a lifetime) at 50 mg per kilogram of body weight. For most of us, this probably translates to about four 12-ounce cans of diet soda or nine 8-ounce glasses of fruit drink made from powder.

Pros:

- Each gram of aspartame has four calories, but it adds almost no calories to foods or drinks as we need only a tiny amount of aspartame to mimic the sweetness of sugar.

- The FDA has repeatedly evaluated aspartame use in food and beverages since the sweetener was first approved in 1981. There have been about 200 studies over 40 years.

- In 1996, the FDA approved its use as a general-purpose sweetener in foods and beverages.

- In 1985, the AMA's Council on Scientific Affairs concluded that "available evidence suggests that consumption of aspartame by normal humans is safe and is not associated with serious adverse health effects."

- Use of aspartame within the FDA guidelines appears safe for pregnant women.

Cons:

- Aspartame cannot be consumed by people born with a condition called phenylketonuria. They cannot metabolize the amino acid phenylalanine and need to eliminate it completely from their diet.

- Aspartame breaks down in liquids that are exposed to heat, so you can't bake or cook with it.

- Some people claim they have had allergic reactions to aspartame, ranging from skin reactions to respiratory problems, but this has been difficult to confirm in studies.

- Some people have reported central nervous system side effects, such as headaches, dizziness, and mood changes, after consuming aspartame. But after reviewing 600 of these complaints, the Center for Disease Control concluded there was no association. (The Environmental Nutrition newsletter later reported that the CDC was leaving open the possibility that a small group of people may be sensitive to aspartame.)

Acesulfame-K (Sunette or Sweet One, often paired with Splenda in diet beverages)

Acesulfame-K (the "K" refers to mineral potassium) is 200 times sweeter than sugar. It is approved by the FDA as a tabletop sweetener and an additive to desserts, confections, and alcoholic beverages.

Pros:

- It doesn't increase the risk of cancer, according to government agencies.
- It doesn't affect blood sugar levels.
- It can be used in cooking and baking.
- It isn't broken down by the body during digestion and is excreted from the body unchanged.
- Combining it with other artificial sweeteners can increase the overall sweetness and decrease the bitter taste.
- The use of acesulfame-K within FDA guidelines appears safe for pregnant women.

Cons:

- When used on its own, this sweetener can have a bitter taste.
- The Washington-based consumer group Center for Science in the Public Interest believes the safety tests on acesulfame-K were poorly conducted and did not properly assess the sweetener's cancer-causing potential.

Sugar Alcohols (sorbitol, mannitol, maltitol, and xylitol)

These sugar alcohols are found in nature (in plant foods such as fruits and berries) and are also commercially made for use as sweeteners. They are absorbed slowly, and part of them isn't absorbed at all, which is why consuming larger amounts can lead to diarrhea, gas, and bloating. About 50 percent of the sugar alcohols convert to glucose, so keep in mind that they still have an effect on blood sugar, but to a lesser degree than sugar.

Pros:

- Sorbitol has received the "Generally Recognized as Safe" designation from the FDA.

Cons:

- Some people experience a laxative effect if they consume more than 49 grams of sorbitol or more than 19 grams of mannitol. Some people are more sensitive to this effect than others, and these unwelcome side effects might arise with a smaller dose for them. People with IBS will likely be part of this group.

Stevia

Stevia, a plant native to South America that contains natural sweeteners, is the new kid on the block. Native South Americans are thought to have used stevia as a sweetener for hundreds of years. Stevia was originally available as a dietary supplement and wasn't allowed as a food additive until 2008. I personally haven't been too thrilled with the taste of some of the products I've tried sweetened with stevia but it might appeal to others out there.

Special Precautions and Warnings

Pregnancy and breast-feeding: Not enough is known about the use of stevia during pregnancy and breast-feeding. Stay on the safe side and avoid use.

Pros:

- Sweetness not affected by heat.

- Does not spike blood glucose levels.

- Recognized as safe by the FDA. Stevia, and chemicals contained in stevia, including stevioside and rebaudioside A, is likely safe when used as a sweetener in foods. Rebaudioside A has generally recognized as safe (GRAS) status in the U.S. for use as a sweetener for foods. Stevioside has been safely used in research in doses of up to 1500 mg per day for two years.

- There is some question that it might help lower blood sugar levels and possibly treat type 2 diabetes but more research needs to be done on this.

Cons:

- Can have a bitter "licorice" aftertaste, but some say the taste has recently been improved.

- Still relatively new and therefore has not been as extensively studied.

- Some people seem to have a sensitivity to it—some report experiencing bloating or nausea. Others report dizziness, muscle pain, and numbness.

What's the acceptable daily intake (ADI) for your favorite alternative sweetener? Scientific experts establish safe levels of consumption for every no- and low-calorie sweetener used in foods and beverages—the ADI. Here's a summary of the some of this information for you to factor in to your decision of which sweetener works best for you.

No- and low-calorie sweetener	FDA guidelines for ADI	Number of 12-ounce servings to equal the ADI for a 150 (mg/kg) pound person
Acesulfame K	15	20.5
Aspartame	50	18
Saccharin	5	3.5 to 48
Sucralose (Splenda)	5	5.5
Stevia Leaf Extracts	12*	12 to 14

*4 mg/kg/day expressed as steviol equivalents translates into 12 mg/kg/day of steviol glycosides, which are the sweet-tasting components of the stevia leaf extract.

The bottom line on no- and low-calorie sweeteners

Research and experience suggest that diet soft drinks and beverages can have a role helping people with their type 2 diabetes and weight loss. But it isn't a magic bullet either. In other words, don't expect that simply switching to sugar-free products will help you lose weight and keep it off. This should be just one piece of your plan to start living healthy by eating right, avoiding overeating, and exercising as much as possible.

Limited data exists on intakes of individual low- and no-calorie sweeteners, except aspartame, according to the Academy of Nutrition and Dietetics Evidence Analysis Library. Even in the worst case assumption, where aspartame is the only no- or low-calorie sweetener used by the population, the highest level of consumption among adults doesn't even hit 30 percent of the ADI for aspartame. This still isn't justification, in my view, to drink diet beverages all day long.

A recent review on alternative sweeteners summarized that "artificial sweeteners, especially in beverages, can be a useful aid to maintain reduced energy intake and body weight and decrease risk of type 2 diabetes and cardiovascular disease compared with sugars." However, the researchers also reported that long-term intervention trials were still needed (*Curr Opin Clin Nutr Metab Care* 15 [2012]: 597–604).

So, which is best when you want to choose a "diet" or "sugar-free" food or drink? That's really up to you as you weigh the pros and cons of each, but it seems many of the Certified Diabetes Educators I spoke with suggest Splenda or NutraSweet to their patients as the low-calorie sweetener of choice. In my view, the sensible saying "everything in moderation" probably comes into play here as well, no matter which one you choose. Choose your favorite times to enjoy them and then switch to water and unsweetened green tea. Water is still what your body wants and needs most of the time.

Chapter 4

The 10 Food Steps to Freedom

You need to work out an individualized eating plan with your dietitian or Certified Diabetes Educator, because what works best to normalize your blood sugar may be different for someone else. But there are 10 things all people with type 2 diabetes can do to improve their health, reduce their risk of heart disease and other health risks, and make normal blood sugar more likely. Following these 10 steps will bring you one giant step closer to feeling better, having normal blood sugar, and living a longer, healthier life.

Step #1: Count carbohydrates and know your ideal carbohydrate budget per meal.

Every Certified Diabetes Educator I spoke with agreed that it is essential to determine your carbohydrate budget per meal to ensure you are hitting your carbohydrate budget. You can compare your carbohydrate intake at a meal to your blood sugar levels one-and-a-half to two hours after the meal, to get a better idea of how to adjust your carbohydrate budget for that particular meal to achieve normal blood sugar.

It isn't that carbohydrates are bad. It's just that you need to know the amount of carbohydrates your body can tolerate (at different times of the day) given your body, medication, and exercise schedule. Also, keep in mind, many Certified Diabetes

Educators believe it is actually more important to know your carbohydrate budget per meal or snack than it is to know what it is per day.

Your individualized carbohydrate budget

If you are not on insulin, try focusing on keeping the number of carbohydrates consistent throughout the day. If you are on insulin, decide with your Certified Diabetes Educator how many carbohydrates to aim for at specific meals. Create a carbohydrate budget, a certain daily and meal total of grams of carbohydrates. If you go over or under these amounts, you may need to adjust your insulin according to your Certified Diabetes Educator's instructions.

Figuring out your carbohydrate budget

No food is off limits! It's more about learning to spend your carbohydrate budget wisely through the day. One of the reasons to focus on counting grams of carbohydrates is because they have the fastest effect on increasing your blood sugar levels. Your Certified Diabetes Educator or dietitian will consider the following factors when calculating your suggested carbohydrate budget, such as:

- Your weight and height.
- Whether or not weight loss is recommended by your health team.
- When and how much exercise you tend to get. (Physical activity acts a bit like insulin in your body and will help lower your blood sugar.)
- Your diabetes medication or insulin and when you take it.
- Other medical issues, such as elevated blood lipids.

? How low can you go with carbohydrates?

The key for many people with type 2 diabetes, in terms of avoiding high blood sugar with diet, is avoiding those common high-carbohydrate, low-fiber meals. Put another way, this means eating meals with a more moderate number of carbohydrates. This can help some people lose weight and have better blood sugars. It doesn't need to be as low in carbohydrates as the Atkins diet, however, according to Rosemary Yurczyk and other dietitians I spoke with, who work day-to-day helping people with type 2 diabetes. People tend to want to view things as black or white, good or bad. And when the true answer lies in practicing moderation, that becomes the tricky part for many people.

Here are answers to some questions I posed to Certified Diabetes Educator Rosemary Yurczyk, MS, RD, CDE:

(?) What are the guidelines for a carbohydrate budget starting point for people with type 2 diabetes?

Rosemary likes to recommend about 30–60 grams per meal for women and about 60–90 grams per meal for men. This seems like a big range, but the amount that often ends up working for her clients depends on their weight, blood sugar goals, exercise, type of medicine, current eating habits, and so on. This is why working closely with a Certified Diabetes Educator to find your personalized carbohydrate budget is a great idea.

A starting point for women

"If you figure that many women trying to lose weight may need to consume about 1,500 calories per day, and 50 percent of their calories come from carbohydrate, that is about 187 grams of carbohydrate per day or about 60 grams per meal," explains Yurczyk. That's for three meals a day, and, if you are using a four-meal-a-day schedule, it works out to around 47 grams of carbohydrates per meal or snack.

For her patients who want to be on less medication and/or who have severe insulin resistance, Rosemary Yurczyk recommends trying a tad fewer carbohydrates: 40 percent calories from carbohydrates. Given this guideline, our calculations for a 1,500 calories per day benchmark, work out to 150 grams of carbohydrates per day or about 50 grams per meal with three meals a day, or 38 grams of carbohydrates per meal with four meals or snacks a day.

A starting point for men

For a man trying to lose weight, the goal is closer to the 2,000 calorie a day benchmark; 50 percent calories from carbohydrates would translate to about 250 grams of carbohydrates per day, or about 80 grams of carbohydrates per meal for three meals a day. If you are using the four-meal-a-day schedule, it works out to around 60 grams of carbohydrates per meal or snack.

For her male patients that want to be on less medication and/or who have severe insulin resistance, Rosemary Yurczyk recommends trying a little less: 40 percent calories from carbohydrates. Given this guideline, our calculations for a 2000-calories-per-day benchmark work out to 200 grams of carbohydrate per day, or about 66 grams per meal with three meals a day, or 50 grams of carbohydrate per meal with four meals or snacks a day.

A piece of cake or a cup of rice

For the most part, if the number of carbohydrates is the same, a serving of cake is a lot like a serving of rice, pasta, or bread. The effect on your blood sugar will be similar, particularly if it is eaten as part of a meal instead of by itself.

? Is there a certain number of moderate-sized meals per day that seems to work best?

Most of Rosemary's patients still eat three meals a day, plus a snack if needed in the afternoon. The most important thing to Rosemary is that their food is distributed throughout the day and that they are eating about every four hours.

This might look like:

- Breakfast around 7 to 8 a.m.

- Lunch sometime around noon.

- A small afternoon snack between 3 and 4 p.m.

- A light dinner around 6 to 7 p.m.

- Some wonderfully flavored decaf green tea (or other non-calorie or low-cal beverage that you enjoy) around 9 p.m.

? Is morning a problematic time due to higher insulin resistance in the morning? What works best at this time of day?

Increased hormones in the morning seem to increase insulin resistance for people with type 2 diabetes, according to Rosemary. Being vigilant about keeping track of the carbohydrate grams and fiber grams eaten at breakfast and the resultant blood sugar (in a journal) will help people understand what the ideal number of carbohydrate and fiber grams is for them first thing in the morning. This might be a time of day when you need to shoot for the lower number of carbohydrates per meal (50 grams for women and 66 grams for men) and when you really want to reach that per meal fiber goal of around 10 grams of fiber.

? How does fiber fit into one's carbohydrate budget?

You can't talk about carbohydrates and type 2 diabetes, or carbo-hydrates and good health in general, without talking about fiber. Remember how having a good amount of fiber in your meals helps the body better manage the carbohydrate grams you are eating? Well, your carbohydrate budget will also have a fiber budget. Whereas the carbohydrate budget is there to make sure you aren't going over it, the fiber budget is there to make sure you aren't going below it. "I think people are way too low in their fiber intake," notes Rosemary.

Eating about 25 to 30 grams of fiber a day is a challenging but powerful goal, and this amount of fiber will benefit your body more ways than I can count, start-ing with better blood sugar levels and a happier colon. If you are eating four mod-erately sized meals a day, the desirable fiber amount per meal is in the ballpark of seven grams. Now, that's not too, scary is it?

Don't forget to do the math

Because eating more fiber helps the body manage the carbohydrates in the meal better, many dietitians suggest their patients subtract the grams of fiber in the meal from the carbohydrate grams being eaten to give the net amount of car-bohydrate grams.

In other words, if you ate 50 grams of carbohydrates in your meal and the meal also contains seven grams of fiber, your true, or net, number of carbohydrates to subtract from your daily carbohydrate budget would be 43. Make sense?

Two quick tools for carb counting

Tool #1: Check out the one-page carb counting guide I put together on the fol-lowing page. I wanted to make counting as easy as possible. Make a copy of the guide and take it with you when you eat out and use it when you don't have the nutritional information easily available for your meals.

Tool #2: The "Eat What You Love, Love What You Eat with Diabetes Plate" from *www.diabetesandmindfuleating.com* (and the book, *Eat What You Love, Love What You Eat with Diabetes*) can really help some people with diabetes visualize how to put an ideal meal together. I urge you to check this Website out and look at their diagram of the Diabetes Plate. Basically, picture a plate and draw a line down the center from north to south. On the entire left half of the plate, visualize low-carbohydrate vegetables for the meal. On the right hand side, visualize the lower right of the plate for lean protein food choices and the upper right for grains and starchy vegetables (like potatoes and corn). To the right of the plate, next to the grains or starchy vegetables, picture a glass or cup for a possible dairy option and a

General Carbohydrate Counting

15-gram Carbohydrate Servings

Breads & Grains

1 slice of bread
½ of a hamburger or hot dog bun
½ English muffin
½ bagel
6-inch tortilla
2/3 whole wheat pita pocket
1/3 cup cooked pasta
1/3 cup cooked rice
1/3 cup cooked whole grain (like quinoa)
1 cup minimally sweet cold breakfast
cereal (like Cheerios)
½ cup sweetened breakfast cereal
¼ cup granola
½ cup hot oatmeal, unsweetened
2 (4-inch) pancakes

Fruit

1 small piece of fruit
½ of a large piece of fruit (like a banana)
½ cup frozen fruit
½ cup fruit juice
1 ¼ cup high water fruit (like watermelon,
berries and strawberries)

Milk

1 cup nonfat milk
½ cup nonfat chocolate milk
½ cup fruit-flavored yogurt
2/3 cup plain or "lite" yogurt
2 cups lowfat cottage cheese
½ cup ice cream

Toppings

1 tablespoon
syrup, jam, jelly
or honey

Mixed Main Dishes

½ cup casserole
(or similar)
1 cup broth or
tomato-based soup
(not chunky)
½ cup soup chunky
with beans, pasta,
or potato

Beans & Vegetables

1/3 cup cooked beans
½ cup starchy vegetables (corn, potato etc.)
1 ½ cups high water vegetables (broccoli,
cauliflower, zucchini, etc.)
*Raw lettuce is negligible with 2-3 cups
containing 6 grams carbs

Bakery Treats

2 small cookies
2-inch square
brownie cake without
frosting

cup for a fruit option. Even though dairy contains protein, it also can contain varying amounts of lactose or milk sugars, which count as carbohydrates (on the nutrition label they are listed as "sugars"). The upper right side of the plate is where pretty much all of your carbohydrate-containing foods are visually represented.

What about dessert, you ask? If you opt for a dessert that contains carbohydrates, it can take the place of one or more of your carbohydrate choices (the ones in the upper right quarter of your plate).

Putting it all together: quick and healthy meals for people with diabetes

Put the phrase, "I can't eat that—I have diabetes," out of your vocabulary because no food is off limits when you have diabetes. In sensible amounts and as part of a balanced meal, any carbohydrate-containing food can be included. The key is learning how to create a balance in your total meal to produce normal blood sugar after meals, day after day. Use daily testing of blood sugar as an opportunity to learn what is working for you and how your blood sugar is affected by different circumstances.

For most people with diabetes this involves adhering closely to a certain number of carbohydrate grams per meal (about 45–75 grams of carbohydrates eaten three times a day, depending on the person and the meal) and balancing those grams with fiber and protein. Carb-containing foods with fiber and helpful nutrients (vegetables, beans/legumes, whole grains, and whole fruits) generally don't cause blood sugar to rise as high as carbs without fiber. Fiber and protein generally help blunt the rise in blood sugar after a meal. Fat can also play a role in helping normalize blood sugar (if sensible amounts of smart fats—found in nuts, avocado, fish, olives, and so on—are eaten); or fat can contribute to insulin resistance (if higher amounts of saturated fat are eaten).

Suggestions from The American Diabetes Association on diabetes super foods and healthy food choices in general, were considered for the following quick and healthy meal ideas.

Quick and healthy breakfast ideas

Breakfast Wrap

Scramble one egg and two egg whites (or 1/4 cup egg substitute) in a small nonstick frying pan coated with cooking spray. On a microwave-safe plate, spread the eggs down the center of a multigrain or low-carb flour tortilla and top with desired garnishes (such as 1/4 cup chopped tomato, chopped green onions, 1/4 avocado, or 1/8 cup shredded reduced fat cheese) and microwave on high for about 20 seconds to soften tortilla and warm up the filling. Wrap up and enjoy!

    Estimated: carbohydrate: 30 grams, protein: 18 grams, fiber: 6 grams.

High Protein Berry Yogurt Bowl

    Add a cup of plain, nonfat Greek yogurt in a cereal bowl. Stir in a teaspoon of honey and a sprinkle of ground cinnamon if desired. Sprinkle 1/2 cup of frozen or fresh berries over the top and 1/2 cup of whole-grain breakfast cereal of your choice (choose one that adds about 15 grams of carbohydrates and at least 5 grams fiber per 1/2 cup).

    Estimated: carbohydrate: 47 grams, protein: 22 grams, fiber: 10 grams.

PB & J English Muffin

    Toast a whole wheat English muffin and spread one tablespoon of natural-style peanut butter on one side and one tablespoon of less sugar jam on the other side. Enjoy with a whole piece of fruit, like an orange or banana.

    Estimated: carbohydrate: 47 grams, protein: 10 grams, fiber: 7 grams.

Gourmet Cereal Bowl

    Add a cup of your favorite whole grain cereal with about 30 grams of carbohydrates and at least 5 grams of fiber, to a big cereal bowl. Sprinkle 1/2 of fresh or frozen berries or banana slices, and 1/8 cup of toasted nuts (almonds, walnuts, or pecans) over the top. Drizzle 3/4 cup of nonfat milk or soymilk over the top, stir, and enjoy!

    Estimated: carbohydrate: 48 grams, protein: 22 grams, fiber: 15 grams.

French Toast That's Ready When You Are

    French toast freezes well, so make a little extra on the weekends to freeze, then microwave for a special weekday morning breakfast. For one serving, blend together one large egg, one egg white or two tablespoons egg substitute, 1/4-cup nonfat milk or fat-free half and half, 1/2-teaspoon vanilla extract, and 1/4-teaspoon ground cinnamon. Soak about three small or two large slices of whole wheat bread in egg mixture and lightly brown in a nonstick frying pan coated with cooking spray. Top with 1/2 cup fresh or frozen berries or other fruit.

    Estimated: carbohydrate: 60 grams, protein: 21 grams, fiber: 10 grams.

Quick and healthy lunch ideas

Easy Tuna Lunch Salad

Mix a six ounce can of water-packed tuna (drained) with three table-spoons of a light Italian vinaigrette dressing, then add 1/2 cup grape or coarsely chopped tomatoes, 1/8 cup nuts and/or sliced olives, and serve on two cups firmly packed spinach leaves! Enjoy with an ounce of whole grain crackers.

Estimated: carbohydrate: 35 grams, protein: 54 grams, fiber: 6 grams.

Grilled Tomato and Cheese Sandwich with Soup

Heat a nonstick frying pan over medium heat. Coat the pan with cooking spray, lay a slice of whole wheat bread on top, then top with one and a half ounces of reduced fat cheese of your choice and three slices of vine-ripened garden tomatoes. Lay a second piece of whole wheat bread on the top and coat with canola cooking spray. When the underside is golden, flip the sandwich over and lightly brown the other side. Serve with a broth or tomato-based soup with about 10 grams of carbohydrate, per one cup serving.

Estimated: carbohydrate: 60 grams, protein: 27 grams, fiber: 8 grams.

3-Minute Bean & Cheese Burrito

Lay a multi-grain or low carb flour tortilla burrito on a paper towel and cook on HIGH for about 30 seconds or until it's soft. Sprinkle 1/3 cup of shredded reduced-at Monterey Jack or cheddar over the top of the tortilla. Spoon 1/2 cup of no-fat canned refried beans (or similar) evenly in center, along with one tablespoon of fat-free sour cream, one tablespoon of salsa, and some chopped green onion or tomato (as desired). Roll it up into a burrito and microwave until it is hot throughout.

Estimated: carbohydrate: 50 grams, protein: 24 grams, fiber: 10 grams.

Lunchtime Pasta Salad

Leftover multigrain cooked pasta from dinner can become tomor-row's lunch just by tossing one cup of the leftover pasta with one cup of cooked green or cruciferous vegetables of your choice, an ounce of cubed or shredded part-skim mozzarella or 1/2 cup leftover grilled seafood/chicken/lean beef, plus chopped green onions, tomatoes, and sliced olives (if desired). Sprinkle a tablespoon of toasted pine nuts or walnuts over the top along with about two tablespoons of light vinaigrette. Toss and enjoy! This keeps well if you are bringing it to work—keep it in the refrigerator.

Estimated: carbohydrate: 54 grams, protein: 21 grams, fiber: 10 grams.

Turkey Avocado Wrap

Top a multigrain or low-carb tortilla, flatbread, or Naan bread with a tablespoon of basil or sundried tomato pesto or olive tapenade (available in jars), then top with a few slices of roasted turkey, one ounce of reduced-fat provolone (or similar), and about four avocado slices, spinach leaves, and tomato slices if desired. Roll up and wrap in foil or plastic wrap and chill until needed.

Estimated: carbohydrate: 30 grams, protein: 32 grams, fiber: 8 grams.

Quick and healthy dinner ideas

Vegetarian or Turkey Simple Salsa Chili

Brown 1/2 pound ground lean turkey or one pound sliced mushrooms with 1/2 onion (chopped) and 1 teaspoon minced garlic in a medium nonstick saucepan coated with a tablespoon of extra virgin olive oil. Add one cup of bottled marinara sauce of choice and one cup prepared or bottled salsa of choice, a 15-ounce can of black or kidney beans (drained), plus chili powder, oregano and ground cumin to taste if desired. Cover and bring to boil. Lower heat and simmer for 20 minutes. This will make three servings. Enjoy each serving with a cup of fruit salad.

Estimated: carbohydrate: 43 grams, protein: 22 grams, fiber: 12 grams.

Fruit and Walnut Chicken Dinner Salad

Cut a leftover grilled boneless, skinless chicken breast into slices (or use a pre-sliced seasoned chicken breast available from a couple of brands) and toss with three or four cups of dark green lettuce, one cup of fresh or frozen berries or a sliced pear or apple, 1/4 cup toasted walnuts or pecans, two tablespoons blue cheese, and two tablespoons of light balsamic vinaigrette or light raspberry vinaigrette.

Estimated: carbohydrate: 27 grams, protein: 37 grams, fiber: 12 grams.

Teriyaki Salmon Dinner

(Substitute another type of fish or skinless/boneless chicken breast or thigh if desired.)

Start cooking steamed brown rice (available in the frozen food section in some stores) and begin heating the oven/toaster-oven broiler. Line a pie plate with foil and place salmon filets or steaks on top. Top each piece of fish with two teaspoons of bottled teriyaki sauce. Broil about 6-inches from the broiler for about four minutes. Flip the fish over and spread one tablespoon of the drippings on top of each piece and broil until the fish is cooked throughout. Serve with 3/4 cup of steamed brown rice and a cup of steamed green or cruciferous vegetables.

Estimated: carbohydrate: 42 grams, protein: 29 grams, fiber: 5 grams.

Mushroom Spaghetti Dinner

Start boiling whole grain spaghetti noodles following directions on the package. Sauté a cup of sliced mushrooms (any type) and one and a half teaspoons of olive oil per person in a medium nonstick saucepan. Pour in 3/4 cup of marinara sauce per serving, cover the saucepan, and bring to a boil. Reduce the heat to a simmer and cook for 10 minutes. Serve a serving of the mushroom marinara with 3/4 cup of whole grain cooked pasta and add a garden salad to complete the meal (two cups of spinach or romaine lettuce, 1/4 cup of kidney or garbanzo beans, a few olives, plus assorted vegetables, such as sliced cucumber and carrot, all topped with a tablespoon or two of light vinaigrette).

Estimated: carbohydrate: 60 grams, protein: 18 grams, fiber: 9 grams.

There's weight-loss magic in the food diary

Is there magic in keeping a food diary? One study found it can double a person's weight loss! The researchers discovered that the more food records people kept, the more weight they lost. Published in the August 2008 issue of *American Journal of Preventive Medicine*, the study adds more evidence to the notion that the simple act of writing down what they eat encourages people to consume fewer calories. This is an added bonus for people with diabetes who are also trying to trim off a few extra pounds (Hollis, J. F. et al. "Weight Loss During the Intensive Intervention Phase of the Weight-Loss Maintenance Trial." *American Journal of Preventative Medicine* 35, 2: 118–126).

Most of the commercial food diaries available leave a space only to tabulate grams of carbohydrate. I designed the following A Day at a Glance chart to help you tabulate grams of carbohydrates, plus grams of fat and fiber if desired. Knowing the grams of fat and fiber helps complete the picture for many people with diabetes. You might find that it's the really high-fat meals that cause you trouble, or you might find that a certain number of fat grams, especially if they are smart fats, seem to help normalize your blood sugar. You might discover that your blood sugar levels are better when your meal/snack has a certain number of fiber grams.

The following A Day at a Glance chart includes a space to record how hungry you were when you ate. There is a space to record your blood sugar, your medication, the minutes, and when you exercised. All this information will help you and your dietitian or diabetes educator fine-tune your eating plan.

A Day at a Glance

Blood Sugar Measurements
6 a.m.:
8 a.m.:
10 a.m.:
12 p.m.:
 2 p.m.:
4 p.m.:
6 p.m.:
8 p.m.:
10 p.m.:
12 a.m.:
2 a.m.:

Insulin or Oral Measurements
(record units or number of tablets taken at what times)
6 a.m.:
8 a.m.:
10 a.m.:
12 p.m.:
2 p.m.:
4 p.m.:
6 p.m.:
8 p.m.:
10 p.m.:
12 a.m.:
2 a.m.:

Activity (minutes)
6 a.m.:
8 a.m.:
10 a.m.:
12 p.m.:
2 p.m.:
4 p.m.:
6 p.m.:

8 p.m.:
10 p.m.:
12 a.m.:
2 a.m.:

Meals/Snacks	Day:_____			Date: ___/___/___
meal/snack	carbs	fat	fiber	hunger level
meal/snack	carbs	fat	fiber	hunger level
meal/snack	carbs	fat	fiber	hunger level
meal/snack	carbs	fat	fiber	hunger level

(*Hunger level: 4=very hungry, 3=moderately hungry, 2=somewhat hungry, 1=not really hungry)

Step #2: Switch to smart carbohydrates and emphasize low-glycemic-load foods.

It isn't just about the quantity of carbs, it's the quality of the carbs that matters to people threating or preventing type 2 diabetes.

Is the glycemic index, or GI (essentially, a number that says how much your blood sugar rises after you eat a particular food that contains carbohydrates), really the be-all, end-all to nutrition and health? Well, not exactly.

High-GI foods, such white bread and white rice, give you a quick blood sugar boost that also fades quickly, leaving you hungry again. Lower GI foods, such as whole grains, produce, and beans, keep you feeling full longer, because they cause your blood sugar levels to rise more slowly.

I call the glycemic index a work in progress, because, though it is certainly one tool that can be considered when making food choices, it's not the only means to measure what you eat. That's because it's based on how blood sugar rises in response to one particular food, such as carrots or rice. But we don't sit down to just a bowl of carrots or a plate of rice, do we? We eat foods together, as dishes and meals. The presence of fat or fiber in a meal also influences how quickly our bodies metabolize the carbohydrates. So do some other factors, such as how long noodles are cooked, or how finely the grain is ground. For example, slightly under-cooked noodles are absorbed more slowly and have a lower GI, and the more finely a grain is ground, the more quickly its carbohydrates are absorbed.

Here's where the controversy kicks in. Researchers and experts continue to disagree on whether low-GI foods lead to weight loss, lower blood sugar levels, and/or a reduced risk of heart disease and cancer compared with high-GI foods.

After reviewing the existing research, the American Institute for Cancer Research concluded. "Due to insufficient evidence of clinical efficiency and persistent methodological concerns regarding how glycemic index values are determined, AICR cautions the public not to make dietary changes based solely on this interesting but still unproven concept." Enter a potentially more useful tool: the glycemic load.

The better way to measure

The glycemic load (GL) is like the glycemic index in that the lower the number, the better the blood glucose response is predicted to be. But GL values allow comparisons of the likely glycemic effect of realistic serving sizes of the foods. So, though carrots tend to have a somewhat high glycemic index, the glycemic load is actually low because it factors in the grams of carbohydrates for a realistic serving size. It's the glucose load that was recently shown in a meta-analysis to be related to consistently lower type 2 diabetes risk in person consuming lower glucose load diets (AMJlinNutr 2013, 97: 584-596).

What this means is that the glycemic index tells you how quickly a particular carbohydrate in food makes your blood sugar rise, but it doesn't take into account how many carbohydrates are found in a typical serving. That means that some healthy but relatively low-carbohydrate foods—such as carrots, watermelon, or popcorn—end up with a high GI number.

The glycemic load, meanwhile, takes the number of carbohydrates per serving into consideration along with the food's glycemic index. To find a food's glycemic load, you multiply its GI value by number of available carbohydrates per serving.

?

What influences the glycemic load and glycemic index?

Many factors help determine your body's glycemic response to a particular food, including:

- **Physical form, such as a whole apple vs. applesauce:** Mashing foods tends to give them a higher glycemic index/load.

- **Ripeness:** The riper the fruit, the higher its glycemic index.

- **Fiber:** Particularly viscous fiber, a type of soluble fiber found in oats, barley, and other foods. Generally, the higher the fiber, the lower the glycemic index/load.

- **Acidity:** The higher a food's acidity, the lower its glycemic index/load.

- **Processing:** The more processed or refined a food, generally, the higher its glycemic index/load will be. When a grain is in a more "whole" form, your body's digestive enzymes have a tougher time breaking it down, which lowers the glycemic response to it. There are some notable exceptions: pasta, and parboiled and basmati rice tend to have lower glycemic indexes, especially if they're not overcooked.

- **Whether protein and fat were eaten with the food:** The presence of high amounts of protein and fat will decrease the glycemic index/load.

The bottom line on glycemic load and glycemic index

I always look for the bottom line, and in the case of glycemic load, it tends to lead you to less-processed types of carbohydrate-rich foods, such as vegetables, fruits, whole grains, beans, and legumes. The truth is that there is plenty of evidence that a mostly plant-based diet can reduce your risk of diseases such as cancer, heart disease, and diabetes. And these foods tend to have lower glycemic index numbers. But we have yet to determine whether a low-glycemic-index diet is really what helps prevent disease, or whether this effect comes mostly from eating a healthful variety of foods.

Glycemic load and index values for common foods

Here are glycemic index (GI) and glycemic load (GL) values for some common foods (Diabetes Care Dec. 2008 vol. 31, number 12, pages 2281-2283). Keep in mind that GI/GL is just one tool. Other aspects of food (such as vitamin, mineral, fiber, and phytochemical content) are also extremely valuable to our health. This table uses glucose as the reference for glycemic index (glucose = 100). In many cases I took an average of several values from the medical journal table and used American data if available. Foods that meet the guidelines for "low glycemic index" and "low glycemic load" will be in BOLD in the table below.

GL: Low = 1-10
    Mid = 11-19
    High = 20+

GI: Low = 1-55
    Mid = 56-69
    High = 70-100

FOOD	GI	GL
BEVERAGES		
Milk, whole	40	4
Milk, skim	37	6
Gatorade, orange	89	13
Poweraid, orange	65	13

JUICES		
Apple, unsweetened	41	12
Grapefruit, unsweetened	48	9
Orange, unsweetened	57	15
BREADS		
Bagel, white	72	25
Baguette, plain	95	14
Rye, light	68	10
Whole wheat bread	67	8
BREAKFAST CEREALS		
All-Bran	50	12
Bran Chex	58	11
Cheerios	74	15
Corn Chex	83	21
Cornflakes	92	24
Cream of Wheat	66	17
Crispix	87	22
Golden Grahams	71	18
Grape-Nuts	67	13
Oats, one-minute	66	17
Oat bran, raw	59	3
Rice Chex	89	23
Rice Krispies	82	22
Shredded Wheat	83	17
Total	76	17

GRAINS

Barley, pearl	22	9
Buckwheat	51	15
Bulgur, cracked wheat, boiled	46	12
Corn, sweet, cooked	57	19
Couscous, boiled 5 min.	61	21
Millet	71	26

RICE

Long grain white boiled 15 min.	58	23
Brown rice, steamed	50	17

DAIRY

Ice cream	62	7
Ice cream, chocolate	68	10
Milk, whole	40	4
Yogurt, flavored lowfat approx.	51	15
Yogurt, fruit, "light" approx.	45	5

FRUIT

Apple	40	6
Banana	51	13
Cherries	22	3
Dates, dried	103	42
Grapefruit	25	3
Grapes	43	7
Kiwifruit	47	6
Mango	41	8
Orange	48	5
Peach	28	4

Pear	33	4
Pineapple	51	8
Plum	24	3
Raisins	66	28

VEGETABLES

Broccoli, steamed	6	1
Spinach, steamed	6	1
Green peas, frozen	39	3
Sweet corn, boiled	57	13
Carrots, boiled approx.	60	4
Potato, baked	82	27
Sweet potato	48	16
Yam	51	18

LEGUMES/BEANS

Black-eyed peas	50	15
Garbanzo beans	33	10
Kidney beans	23	6
Lentils, red	26	5
Pinto beans	39	10

PREPARED/CONVENIENCE FOODS

Cheese tortellini	50	10
Fish sticks	38	7
French fries, from frozen	75	22
Pizza, cheese	60-80	16-22

PASTA		
Macaroni, boiled 5 minutes	45	22
Spaghetti, boiled 5 minutes	38	18
SNACK FOODS		
Corn chips	74	21
Crackers, soda	74	12
Crackers, stoned wheat thins	67	11
Crackers, rye crisp bread	63	11
Peanuts	13	1

? Do beans/legumes have super powers?

When was the last time you ate beans? Maybe the last time you ate Mexican food? There is a whole lot more to beans than burritos. Beans offer a unique food package contributing both types of fiber, carbohydrates, and protein, along with vitamins, minerals, and assorted phytochemicals (plant compounds).

Beans are a great food to add to a meal or snack because they may help improve blood sugar control in people with type 2 diabetes. How do beans do this? It's the whole nutritional bean package that makes this happen. The plant protein and fiber in beans slow digestion (releasing carbohydrates into the bloodstream slowly and steadily), which can help lessen the rise in blood sugar. The protein may help stimulate the release of insulin after the meal, while the protein and fiber also enhance the feeling of fullness during and after the meal to keep you feeling satisfied longer.

A half-cup of beans offers:
- 22 grams of carbohydrates.
- 8 grams of fiber.
- 8 grams of protein.
- Key vitamins (folic acid, B vitamins).
- Key minerals (such as potassium, magnesium, calcium and iron).

Any questions? Bottom line: use beans because they have super powers!
Bean tips:

- Save time using canned beans. Just drain and rinse them and you are good to go. Rinsing can help remove some of the gas-producing substances in beans as well as some of the sodium. You can also buy the lower-sodium variations of canned beans.

- Some beans are even available frozen such as edamame, fava beans, and black-eyed peas.

- Order beans in restaurants either on the side or choose entrees that feature beans.

- Add beans to green or grain salads (edamame, kidney, garbanzo, and black beans work well).

- Hummus is a nice filling snack made with garbanzo beans and served with whole-wheat pita bread, crackers, or raw veggies. You can also make hummus with fava beans or edamame (for a green hummus).

- Hummus also makes a great spread on your bread when making sandwiches (replacing mayonnaise or other creamy spreads).

- When making a Mexican entrée, replace half of the meat in the filling with beans (pinto and black beans work very well).

- Add beans to soups and stew—it will make them more filling (lentils, garbanzo, kidney, black beans, and edamame work well).

- Add beans to your favorite casserole. All beans work.

Check out the new recipes in Chapter 5 that feature beans and legumes.

Intact whole grains are ideal

Switching to whole grains every chance you get is certainly a big step in the right direction because whole grain breads and cereals have fiber and nutrients you don't get with processed grains and products. But even better is adding intact whole grains to your daily diet—they are digested more slowly, and add fiber, important nutrients (some include protein), and plant compounds along with grams of carbohydrates.

Intact whole grains are grains in their mainly "whole" form being cooked and eaten like when you cook barley, brown or wild rice, or steel cut or old fashioned oats. But there are some awesome ancient whole grains that you should try to incorporate as well. Have you heard of quinoa, kamut, buckwheat, spelt, or millet? These are just a handful of the intact whole grains that are now available in stores everywhere or online. Check out the recipes with intact whole grains in Chapter 5!

The whole grain that is almost a complete protein—quinoa

Once considered the "gold of the Incas," quinoa is thought to have been an important food for more than 6,000 years—Incan tribes in the Andes Mountains cultivated it, for example. Knowing that long and rich history kind of makes you want to try it, right?

I tried black quinoa in a restaurant, which at first glance looked like poppy seeds on steroids, but the quinoa grains were tender and complemented the tasty tofu entrée I had with it. Newly inspired, I then cooked up some of the quinoa sample I had at home. I threw some into my rice cooker with chicken broth (two cups per cup of dry quinoa) and pressed the "brown rice" setting. It worked like a charm and couldn't have been easier.

Why try quinoa? Here are five nutritional reasons:
- Quinoa is a unique grain in that it has all nine essential amino acids, making it a complete protein.
- Quinoa is higher in protein than similar grains (7 grams protein per 1/4 cup dry).
- Quinoa is notably rich in polyphenols (phytochemicals known for their potentially protective antioxidant activity) as compared to other grains.
- Each serving also adds 3 grams of fiber and 10 percent of the daily value for iron.
- Quinoa is gluten-free.

Action item: Cook quinoa as you would brown rice (2 parts water or broth of your choice to 1 cup of dry quinoa) and you can substitute it for rice, bulgur, or cracked wheat in most recipes to make dishes like pilafs or tabbouleh. I like making entrée salads with quinoa, adding vegetables and tofu, edamame, fish, or chicken.

The smart carb bonus—fiber!

Fiber is the part in plant foods that humans can't digest. Because we can't digest it, it makes it all the way through the mouth to the stomach, then through the small and large intestines without being absorbed, and out the other end. But even though it isn't absorbed, it does all sorts of great stuff for our bodies.

Research shows that fiber helps reduce the rapid rise in blood sugar that tends to take place after eating foods containing carbohydrates. It does this by slowing down their digestion. This could help blunt the impact of eating carbohydrates on people at risk for diabetes.

There are two types of fiber. There is insoluble fiber, which doesn't dissolve in water and contributes "roughage" or "bulk" to our intestinal tract. It acts as a scrubber, pushing food along and helping to clean the intestinal wall as it passes through. This is the type of fiber that is thought to help treat and prevent diverticulosis (a condition in which small pouches form in the colon wall and can become infected) and is linked to reducing the risk of constipation and colon cancer. It is possible that the fiber latches onto potential carcinogens within the intestines and carries them out of the body.

The second type of fiber is particularly important if you have type 2 diabetes: soluble fiber. Soluble fiber is different from the other type of fiber because it dissolves in water and becomes almost gel-like. Soluble fiber does appear to lower total serum cholesterol and LDL cholesterol levels (the higher your cholesterol levels, the more it will help lower it). It also helps regulate blood sugar. Because soluble fiber helps regulate blood sugar, high-fiber diets have been reported to:

- Lower postprandial blood sugar. (It may even improve glucose control in the meals immediately following.)
- Decrease glucose in the urine.
- Decrease insulin needs and increase tissue sensitivity to insulin.
- Reduce levels of atherosclerosis-promoting blood lipids.

It is soluble fiber, in particular, that may help lessen the potential increase in blood triglycerides and other blood fats seen in some diabetics on a high-carbohydrate diet.

One study showed that a high-fiber eating plan reduced insulin requirements by 75 percent in people with type 2 diabetes. Some people were able to get off insulin completely. There is one catch—soluble fiber helps lower your glucose level *after* meals, and, to a lesser extent, upon wake-up. But this is still super-helpful because we spend most of our 24-hour day in a post-meal state, right? How much total fiber are we talking about? A stiff daily dose of about 30 grams of fiber.

In another study on men with diabetes, this one from UCLA, a combination of a higher-fiber, low-fat diet resulted in significant reductions in fasting glucose and insulin levels as well as in body mass index and all serum lipids (*Diabetes Research Clinical Practice* [September 2006] 73(3): 249–59).

How much fiber do we need to get our heart disease prevention benefits? In one study, men who ate more than 25 grams of fiber per day (soluble and insoluble), reduced their risk of heart disease by 36 percent, compared to men who ate less than 15 grams of fiber daily. Does this sound impossible? With the right tips and recipes, and maybe a small hill of beans, some of us can hit this mark on most days.

? *How does soluble fiber work its magic?*

Fiber slows down the absorption of other nutrients eaten at the same meal, including carbohydrates. This slowing down may help prevent peaks and valleys in your blood sugar. It has also been suggested that higher-fiber meals improve your body sensitivity to insulin, so it may reduce the insulin requirements in insulin-treated type 2 diabetics.

As it passes through the intestines, soluble fiber holds onto anything it can and carries it out of the body. One of the things we know it holds onto is bile (digestive juices that the body produces using cholesterol from the body), so our body has to keep making more bile, using more cholesterol. This reduces blood cholesterol levels. Every body responds differently, but, for some people, combining soluble fiber with a low-fat eating plan can mean serum cholesterol reductions of 50 points or more.

Getting fiber at almost every meal

The problem is that the typical American diet is anything but high in fiber. "White" grain is the American mode of operation; we eat a muffin or bagel made with white flour in the morning, have our hamburger on a white bun, and then have white rice with our dinner. The more refined, or "whiter," the grain-based food, the lower the fiber.

To get some fiber into almost every meal takes effort. Start by:

- Eating plenty of fruits and vegetables. Just eating five servings a day of fruits and vegetables (something we should do anyway) will get you to about five grams of soluble fiber. See Step #6 for more on fruits and vegetables.
- Including some beans and bean products in your diet. A half cup of cooked beans will add about two grams of soluble fiber to your day.
- Switching to whole grains whenever possible, particularly intact whole grains such as quinoa, barley, kamut, and buckwheat groats, and so on.

Thanks to all the wonderful whole-grain blend pastas now on the market, higher-fiber pasta is now a way of life in the Magee house. Just switch where you can but know that the more you switch from refined-grain products to the higher-fiber whole-grain foods, the better off you will be with your health in general and, most likely, with your diabetes.

? *Where can you find soluble fiber?*

Most plant foods contain some insoluble fiber and some soluble fiber. About one-quarter to one-third of the total amount of fiber in plants is the soluble type, but some plant foods have more than others. The following foods are some of the richest sources of soluble fiber.

- **Beans:** One-half cup cooked kidney beans, butter beans, canned baked beans, black beans, navy beans, lentils, pinto beans, great northern beans, chick peas or garbanzo, split peas, and lima beans. Some of the soluble fiber dissolves in the liquid of canned beans, so if you are making a soup or stew, just stir the liquid in.

- **Oats and oat bran:** One-half cup dry oat bran contributes three grams of soluble fiber, and one cup of cooked oatmeal contains about two grams of soluble fiber. One packet of instant oatmeal contributes one gram of soluble fiber.

- **Barley:** This grain has been enjoyed in other parts of the world for hundreds of years. In America, you sometimes find it in soups. Even pearl barley, which has been milled, still contributes 1.8 grams of soluble fiber per three-fourths-cup cooked serving.

- **Some fruits:** Apples; mangos; plums; kiwis; pears; blackberries; strawberries; raspberries; peaches; citrus fruits, including oranges and grapefruits (you'll get the most soluble fiber if you include the "pulp" and membranes, dividing the fruit into sections); and dried fruits including dried apricots, prunes, and figs.

- **Some vegetables:** Artichokes, celery root, sweet potato, parsnip, turnip, acorn squash, potato with skin, Brussels sprouts, cabbage, green peas, broccoli, carrots, French-style green beans, cauliflower, asparagus, and beets.

- **Psyllium seed products:** One rounded kitchen teaspoon of most psyllium products will give you about three grams of soluble fiber.

Top 20 Viscous (Soluble Fiber) Foods	Soluble Fiber	Total Fiber	Calories	Protein (g)
Passion fruit, purple, 1 cup	12.3	25	229	5
Guava, fresh, 1 cup	4.5	9	112	4
Navy Beans, cooked 1/2 cup	2.8	9.5	127	8
Refried beans, fat-free, 1/2 cup	2.5	6	110	7
Cranberry beans, cooked, 1/2 cup	3.4	9	120	8
Cheerios cereal, 1 1/2 cups	2.9	4.5	165	5
Kidney beans, red, cooked, 1/2 cup	2.7	7	112	8
French beans, cooked 1/2 cup	2.6	8	114	6
Split green peas, cooked, 1/2 cup	2.5	8	116	8
Asian pears, fresh, 1	2.4	4	51	1

Life cereal, plain, 1 1/2 cups	2.3	4	239	6
Rye crisp bread crackers, 2 ounces	2.1	9	207	5
Pinto beans, canned, 1/2 cup	2.1	6	103	6
Black beans, canned, 1/2 cup	2.1	8	113	8
Orange, fresh medium, 1	2.1	3	62	1
Pink grapefruit, fresh, 1	2.1	3	91	1
Parsnips, fresh slices, 1 cup	2	7	100	2
Oats, rolled old fashioned, 1/2 cup	2	4	150	5
Mung beans, fresh, 1/4 cup	2	9	179	12
Savoy cabbage cooked, 1 cup	2	4	35	3

Give it time and lots of water

Most people's bodies seem to adjust to more fiber in their diet within about six weeks. While your body is adjusting, you may notice a little uninvited gas. To minimize the side effects (diarrhea, abdominal pain, and flatulence) increase your fiber *slowly* and drink plenty of water (which you should be doing anyway). Soluble fiber, especially, absorbs water like a sponge, so drink up!

You can also try Beano or Beanzyme pills, which can be found in your local drugstore or on the Internet. They contain an enzyme that, when taken along with beans, cabbage, broccoli, and other vegetables, helps reduce the side effects. For a handful of great bean recipes, see Chapter 6. For lists of higher-fiber cereals, see Chapter 7.

The high-fiber bonus for calorie watchers

Both fiber types help us feel fuller faster when they are part of the meal, discouraging overeating. When people eat meals higher in fiber, they tend to eat less. One study found that people ate smaller lunches after eating high-fiber breakfasts. Why? Fiber lowers insulin, and insulin helps stimulate your appetite. And fiber seems to help make you feel full.

There is also some evidence that fiber can help cut calories by blocking the digestion of some of the fat, protein, or carbohydrates eaten at the same time. Either way, eating fiber is a good thing if you are overweight.

Step #3: Model the Mediterranean diet

The traditional Mediterranean diet may not just be good for the heart; there is some evidence suggesting it may also help people prevent and treat type 2 diabetes and prevent weight gain. Keep in mind the Mediterranean diet is more than a list of foods—it's a lifestyle. It includes slowing down and enjoying meals, usually with friends and family, and eating foods that are local and in-season rather than processed food products.

What is the Mediterranean way of eating?

- Meals are mainly plant based, including whole grains, fruits and vegetables, beans, nuts and seeds, olives, and extra virgin olive oil.

- Use fresh herbs and spices to season food and cut back on adding salt, sugar, and fat for flavor.

- Extra virgin olive oil is used instead of butter and margarine or animal fats.

- Eat fish at least twice a week and focus in general on lean protein sources. Fish often used are salmon, tuna, halibut, herring, sardines, trout, and so on.

- Portions of red meat and poultry are generally small—three ounces or less per serving. Red meat is eaten only a few times a month.

- Low-fat dairy, eggs, and cheese are included but in smaller portions than you might see in American kitchens. Poultry may be eaten about two times a week, and eggs every other day or weekly.

- Saturated fat from red meat and dairy is typically less than eight percent of the total calories consumed.

Obviously, many of the culinary components (described previously) of the Mediterranean diet can be modeled without only eating Mediterranean dishes and only using Mediterranean recipes.

The evidence

You might be even more inspired to adopt many of these culinary cues once you hear the recent research on the Mediterranean diet and type 2 diabetes.

- Close adherence to the Mediterranean diet may improve blood vessel wall function in people with abdominal obesity.

- The Mediterranean diet is a useful tool against cardiovascular disease in part by decreasing inflammatory markers.

- The Mediterranean diet may protect against Metabolic Syndrome in Americans.

- An Italian study showed people with type 2 diabetes who ate a Mediterranean diet (with at least 30 percent calories from fat and no more than 50 percent calories from carbs) were better able to manage their diabetes without medications longer than those eating a low fat diet.

- Adherence to the traditional Mediterranean diet was associated with a reduced risk of developing type 2 diabetes in a couple of studies— even though many participants had other risk factors for type 2 such as higher BMI, a family history of diabetes, or high blood pressure.

- Diets rich in monounsaturated fat may improve lipid profiles and gly-cemic control in people with diabetes, which suggests that monoun-saturated fat may improve insulin sensitivity.
- Two trials suggest extra virgin olive oil may protect against insu-lin resistance and Metabolic Syndrome—and that diets with higher amounts of monounsaturated fat may improve insulin sensitivity (which would directly help people with pre-diabetes or type 2).

Mediterranean-izing American cuisine

Most of us can't drop everything and start eating the traditional Mediterranean way, but we can incorporate many aspects into our American meals and snacks. Remember, it isn't a restrictive diet plan, so be inspired to make the changes that make sense for you such as:

- Fill a big portion of your plate with fruits and vegetables, especially green leafy vegetables.
- Eat more fish and less red meat. When eating out, choose an entrée with plenty of vegetables (or order a side of vegetables in place of fries) and avoid those with cream or butter or lots of cheese. For ex-ample, enjoy the grilled fish with vegetables.
- Opt for whole grains whenever possible, preferably intact whole grains such as quinoa, barley, kamut, oats, and so on. Switch to whole-grain breads and pasta. Many restaurants offer those options now.
- Reach for extra virgin olive oil instead of another vegetable oil, es-pecially when olive oil will enhance or complement other flavors in a dish (vinaigrettes, spreads and dips, sauté dishes). Canola oil is still the best choice, though, for high-temperature cooking or when you want a neutral tasting fat when baking.
- Feature beans, legumes, nuts, and seeds in your meals and snacks. Often, you can decrease the amount of meat used in a dish by adding some beans. Nuts and seeds offer a nice textural change as a garnish in entrees and salads.
- End your meal with a naturally sweet food that provides a serving of fruit, such as fresh purple grapes or a baked apple.
- Enjoy olives (green or black) as accents in entrées, salads, or sand-wiches or set them out on the table as easy appetizers.
- Banish the butter from the table and, instead, dip bread in a blend of tasty extra virgin olive oil with balsamic vinegar and a sprinkle of black pepper, herbs, or garlic.

Step #4: Emphasize heart protective fats and count fat grams for the right balance for your meals and snacks.

You might think food fat is food fat. But there are actually three types of fats in food: saturated fatty acids, polyunsaturated fatty acids, and monounsaturated fatty acids. One of them is better for you than the others. The monounsaturated fats do not seem to promote heart disease, plaque in the arteries, and cancer, as the saturated fats and some of the polyunsaturated fats appear to. It's a no-brainer, then, to start using and eating more monounsaturated fats and definitely less saturated fat.

There are basically two common oils which contain mostly monounsaturated fats: canola oil and olive oil. Both offer additional and different health benefits (you'll find out what those are in the following sections), so I personally use both.

There are certain recipes or foods that I eat that require butter, but only if it is truly the best type of fat for that particular food. Even then, I will use the smallest amount I can. When I can, I switch to canola oil, olive oil, or canola margarine. In most sautéing circumstances, I can use canola or olive oil. In many baking recipes, such as some cakes, muffins, even pie crust, I can switch to canola oil. If the cookie or cake recipe calls for creaming the shortening or butter with sugar, then usually I can use my favorite margarine. See Chapter 7 for more information.

Canola oil

You may have heard that canola is a "good" fat—that it contains mostly monounsaturated fat. You may have even heard that it is one of the few plant sources of omega-3 fatty acids. But how much would you need to consume to get a potentially beneficial dose of omega-3 fatty acids? I asked researchers at Best Foods, which makes Mazola's Canola Oil, to send me the actual fatty acid breakdown for one tablespoon of canola oil. I was delighted to find that just one tablespoon contained about 1.5 grams of omega-3 fatty acids (about the same amount found in 3.5 ounces of cooked salmon). A tablespoon also contains nine grams of omega-9 fatty acids (such as oleic acid, a monounsaturated fat which may reduce the development of breast carcinomas) and seven milligrams of mixed tocopherols (a group of antioxidants which includes vitamin E, also known as alpha-tocopherol).

Canola oil has a neutral flavor and can be heated to high temperatures, so I like to use canola oil in baking and frying recipes.

Extra virgin olive oil

The people in the Mediterranean region have been studied lately because they have surprisingly low rates of heart disease, yet their typical diet can include generous amounts of fat. Their cuisine includes abundant seafood, use of olives and olive oil, fruits, vegetables, beans, and nuts. We now know that all of those foods have health benefits for our body—including olive oil.

Olive oil does not contain omega-3 fatty acids as canola oil does, but the majority of fatty acids in olive oil are still the more beneficial monounsaturated fats; 56 to 83 percent of the fatty acids in olive oil are specifically oleic acid. Canola oil contributes more vitamin E than olive oil, but there is something that olive oil adds to your diet that canola oil doesn't—potentially protective phytochemicals found in olives. Extra virgin olive oil will contain the most helpful phytochemicals because it comes from the first press of the olives. I like to use extra virgin olive oil in my Italian recipes, cold salads, marinades, and vinaigrettes. I even use a light brushing of olive oil on the bread when making grilled cheese sandwiches on whole wheat bread.

Switch to Smart Fats

Avoiding greasy, high-fat food is a no-brainer, but within that healthier way of eating, we can improve our health even further by making smart fat choices. The smart fats are mainly fish omega-3s, plant omega-3s, and monounsaturated fat.

So what does this mean in terms of cooking fat and baking fat choices? Olive oil is highest in monounsaturated fat and it contains some important phytochemicals, but it doesn't contribute any of the plant omega-3s. Canola oil is lowest in saturated fat of the cooking oils and contains an impressive amount of monounsaturated fat and contributes the most plant omega-3s of the vegetable oils.

Monounsaturated fats help reduce the risk of heart disease, especially if they replace saturated or trans fat in the foods we eat. They reduce blood pressure and LDL (bad) cholesterol and may help increase HDL (good) cholesterol. If a diet high in monounsaturated fat is combined with eating fewer carbohydrates, it can also improve insulin sensitivity. Some high monounsaturated fat foods are olive oil, canola oil, peanut oil, hazelnut oil, almonds and almond oil (and some other nuts), and avocados.

Omega-3 fatty acids, especially from fish, may help decrease blood clotting, decrease abnormal heart rhythms, reduce triglycerides, and promote normal blood pressure. Plant omega-3s are also helpful, because your body can convert a small amount of the plant omega-3s into the fish omega-3s. Plus, there is some evidence that plant omega-3s lower heart disease risk as well, through different processes than fish omega-3s. It is also possible that omega-3s help to lower cancer risk; scientists are investigating this area as well. Omega-3s seem to have anti-inflammatory action within body tissues, and some researchers suggest getting more omega-3s to reduce the risk of inflammatory diseases.

? Should you count fat grams?

It is helpful for some people with diabetes to count fat grams, because the issue of food fat for most people with type 2 diabetes can be a little tricky. The only way to know what level of fat grams works best for you at what time of day is to count them every now and then. Take a look at your food diary and see what level of fat tends to produce better blood sugar at certain times of day.

Everybody is different, but most people with type 2 diabetes handle carbohydrates better when they are eaten alongside some protein and smart fat. Fat helps lower the blood glucose response to the other foods it is eaten with. So some fat is definitely a good thing—especially if it is one of the more protective types of fats (monounsaturated fat, omega-3). What we are really talking about is a balancing act—pairing your carbohydrate-rich foods (breads, grains, starches, fruits, sweets) with foods that contribute some protein and fat.

It's a good idea, when you are trying to figure out which foods and food combinations you do best with, to count fat grams along with carbohydrate grams. For many people with type 2 diabetes, meals that are too high in fat (especially saturated and animal fats) can have terrible consequences on after-meal blood sugar. In some people, meals high in animal fats make the body very resistant to insulin. Meals such as a sausage and eggs breakfast or your typical pepperoni and sausage pizza can be a blood glucose nightmare.

Cooking with the right fats

If a recipe calls for vegetable oil, just use canola oil. If it calls for vegetable oil and you think the flavor of olive oil would complement the dish and the oil doesn't need be heated to a high temperature (olive oil starts smoking and breaking down at higher temperatures), then you can even use extra virgin olive oil instead. But what about the recipes that call for shortening, stick butter, or margarine?

Sometimes I still use butter because that truly is the best fat for that recipe. I just cut it down as far as I can (substituting in other high flavor/high moisture ingredients). But if butter isn't essential to the recipe, and your original recipe calls for beating the butter, margarine, or shortening in a mixer, usually with sugar and eggs, you can switch to a margarine that lists liquid canola oil as the first ingredient and contains around eight grams of fat per tablespoon. Sometimes you can get away with beating part canola oil and part fat-free cream cheese or sour cream in place of the original fat. If you are just sautéing something in a pan, you can easily switch to canola or olive oil, and you can probably use less than the amount suggested in the original recipe, especially if you are using a nonstick pan.

Start collecting recipes that your family likes that call for olive or canola oil. I made up a reduced-fat pie crust recipe that uses canola oil. I now use salad dressings that contain canola or olive oil for my vinaigrette-dependent recipes (such as green salad and pasta salad). These are the kinds of changes you can start making right now.

Step #5: Keep saturated fat, trans fat, and cholesterol low.

If monounsaturated fat is now "in," then saturated and trans fats are definitely "out." You'd be hard-pressed to find someone who doesn't know that saturated and trans fat are something Americans need to eat less of. High amounts of saturated fat are clearly associated with heart disease. More specifically, saturated fat has been shown to raise bad cholesterol (LDL) and triglycerides in the blood, and trans fat lowers HDL (good) cholesterol in addition to raising LDL (bad) cholesterol levels. Obviously, eating less saturated and trans fat is good, solid advice. Giving that advice is easy; following it is the tough part—especially here in the United States. Saturated fat is synonymous with typical American food. It's in hamburgers, french fries, pizza, hot dogs, and even apple pie, for goodness' sake.

It doesn't matter whether you find your blood sugar improving with a low or moderate fat eating plan; either way, saturated and trans fat and food cholesterol need to be low. Cholesterol should be limited to 200 to 300 milligrams or less a day, and saturated fat is supposed to contribute no more than seven to 10 percent of the total calories. (For someone eating 1,800 calories a day, that comes to 14 to 20 grams of saturated fat a day.)

The terrible trans fats

The effects of trans fatty acids are unsaturated fatty acids that contain at least one double bond in the "trans" configuration. They occur naturally in low levels in meat and dairy products, but most of the trans fats in the American diet come from trans fats formed during the partial hydrogenation of vegetable oils. This process transforms some of the oil's unsaturated fat into trans fatty acids, which makes them more solid and stable. You'll find trans fats in any cooking or table fats that contain partially hydrogenated fat or oils.

Trans fatty acids are akin to the damaging effects of saturated fat, except trans fats offer a double whammy to your blood lipid profile—in addition to raising your bad cholesterol (LDL) levels, as saturated fat does, trans fats also decrease your good cholesterol (HDL) levels at the same time.

This is one of the reasons why many researchers consider trans fats to be a bigger bad boy than saturated fat. Many researchers suspect that trans fats not only increase your risk of heart disease but may increase the risk of type 2 diabetes, colon cancer, and breast cancer in women.

We should get as little trans fat as possible. Here are a few things to keep in mind with trans fats:

#1 Out goes trans but in comes saturated fat

Food companies and restaurants have been taking partially hydrogenated oils and therefore trans fats out of their products but many have replaced them with saturated fat. Palm oil in particular is being used by food companies because it is naturally saturated and performs similarly to the trans fats of the past. There are a few holdout products in the supermarket with substantial trans fats, so keep a lookout when you are choosing your processed foods: microwave popping corn (4 grams of trans in a serving of Jolly Time Blast O Butter), canned frosting (1.5 grams of trans in a serving), and cookies (2 grams of trans in a serving of Safeway Fudge Sticks).

#2 Look to the label

You can find the amount of trans fat on the nutrition information label, but keep in mind that if a product has less than 0.5 grams of trans fat per serving, they can put "0" on the label. So if you see "partially hydrogenated oil" on the ingredient list and it says "0" for trans fat, it probably has some but it is less than 0.5 grams per serving.

#3 No more than two grams of trans a day

The American Heart Association advises Americans to consume no more than two grams of trans fat per day. That's definitely a best-case scenario. In today's food world, it's easier than you think to eat double or triple the daily two-gram goal in just one meal, especially if you eat a lot of processed food.

#4 Trans in fast food land

Many fast-food chains have also been taking the trans fat out of their fast food items (some chains did this earlier than others) but often they are replaced with saturated fat. The nutrition information provided by the fast food chains will answer that question—just look for the grams of saturated fat along with trans fat. Where are trans still hiding? Here are some fast food options I found with higher amounts of trans fat (as of the publication of this edition):

- Carl's Jr. "made from scratch" biscuits add 6 grams of trans fat while the cinnamon raisin biscuit contains 3.5 grams.

- Some of the 6-dollar burgers at Carl's Jr. contain 2.5 grams of trans.

- Long John Silver's Breaded Clams have seven grams of trans fat per serving.

- Each chicken or fish taco at Long John Silver's contains 4 grams of trans.

- A piece of battered fish or a serving of popcorn shrimp from Long John Silver's is worth about 5 grams of trans fat.

- Sirloin burgers at Jack in the Box contain 2.5 grams of trans each and their Ultimate Cheeseburger contains 3 grams.

Saturated fat sources

One of the biggest contributors of saturated fat and cholesterol in the American diet is the meat group, which includes beef, processed meats, eggs, poultry, and other meats. In general, if you choose leaner meats, use egg substitute in place of half the eggs (a good rule of thumb), and take the skin off poultry, you will lower the amount of saturated fat and cholesterol.

The dairy group is another saturated fat contributor, so select lower-fat dairy options and you are guaranteed less saturated fat and cholesterol.

Saturated fat is found in other common foods, such as butter, ice cream, lard, bacon, anything made with coconut and palm oil, and vegetable oils that have been hydrogenated as is the case with stick margarine and shortening. Many of the packaged foods we buy, such as crackers, cookies, snack foods, frozen fried foods, and pastries, contain hydrogenated oils.

Where to cut cholesterol

Plant foods do not contain cholesterol. Where you find high amounts of fat in animals and animal products, generally cholesterol isn't far behind. Food sources highest in cholesterol are egg yolks, organ meats (especially liver), whole-fat dairy products, and higher-fat meats. There are a few fish sources that are a bit higher in cholesterol, such as shrimp, squid, crab, and lobster, but they are low in fat and saturated fat, so don't worry too much about the occasional shrimp cocktail or calamari you enjoy.

Avoiding organ meats is the easy part. Buying skinless chicken is simple too. And I have personally found it no problem at all to switch to low-fat milk and yogurt, reduced-fat cheese, and fat-free sour cream. The egg substitutes today have come a long way making it easy to use half real eggs and half egg substitute when cooking. Muffins, cakes, quiches, even omelets still turn out terrific.

Keep in mind that some people show big changes in their serum cholesterol after dietary cholesterol and saturated fat have been decreased, whereas others show little change. Blame or thank your genetics. Some people are more sensitive to the cholesterol-raising effects of foods high in saturated fat and cholesterol.

Step #6: Calories do count for many people with type 2 diabetes.

As we can only lose body fat when the calories we burn are greater than the calories we take in with food then, indeed, calories do count. The weight loss can improve or reverse your diabetes and insulin resistance.

Listen to your stomach hunger cues. If you are physically hungry, you should eat. When you are no longer hungry, but comfortable, you should stop eating. But all of this needs to take place while following your carbohydrate budget for each meal. If you are still hungry after eating the amount of food determined by your carbohydrate budget, discuss this with your Certified Diabetes Educator. Check out Step #8 for tips on Mindful Eating and refer back to Chapter 2 for more on the trickiness of energy balance and the myths and truths about obesity and weight loss.

Step #7: Eat more fruits and vegetables.

Starting your meals and snacks with vegetable soup or green salad is a trick I've learned with my family. Research has confirmed that when vegetables are served as a first course, there is a decrease in the total calories eaten during the meal. If you start your meal by enjoying vegetables, they will help fill you up so you won't be as likely to overeat the meat or entrée. Eating at a pizza parlor is a perfect example. While you are waiting for your pizza, relax and enjoy a nice green salad with tomato, kidney beans, and other vegetables, making sure to keep regular dressings (preferably vinaigrettes instead of creamy dressings) to about a tablespoon. You'll find that you won't eat as much pizza. However, if you eat the salad at the same time you eat your pizza, you are less likely to eat the salad.

However, for some people with type 2 diabetes, when fruit is eaten before the meal, it may increase insulin and hunger, thus increase the risk of overeating at the meal.

There are many health reasons to eat more fruits and vegetables, such as high doses of fiber, vitamins and minerals, antioxidants, and phytochemicals; and most are naturally low in fat, sugar, and sodium. Often, we just don't get around to eating enough fruits and vegetables. Most people say it is because they aren't as convenient as snack foods and fast food. Others say they simply aren't in the habit. Well, whatever your reason, the time to change is now.

Making fruits and vegetables more habit-forming

I think we would all eat more fruits and vegetables if we just had a mother taking care of us. We need someone to remember to buy the fruits and vegetables, someone to take the time to turn them into beautiful fruit salads or green salads, snack trays, and garnishes or tasty side dishes to our entrées.

Here are some ways to make fruits and vegetables a little more convenient:

- Pack your desk or car with your favorite dried fruits; they will keep for weeks.
- Buy baby carrots and celery sticks and put them out before dinner.
- Take time once a week to make a large spinach salad or vegetable-fortified lettuce salad, and just store it (without dressing) in an airtight

container. You can have crisp, wonderful salad as a snack or with your lunch or dinner for the next few days.

- Every few days make a point of going to your supermarket and picking out the best-tasting and freshest fruits in season. But don't just buy them; remember you have them, and put them out as a snack for the family. Add a few slices or wedges of fruit to each lunch or dinner plate.

- With a few chops of a knife, you can turn a few pieces of fruit into a beautiful fruit salad. Drizzle lemon, pineapple, or orange juice over the top and toss to coat the fruit with it (the vitamin C helps prevent browning).

- Buy your favorite fruits in the winter—just buy them frozen or canned in juice or light syrup.

- Stock your refrigerator at work and home with your favorite fruit juices (make sure they are 100-percent juice), the pulpier the better. You can often buy them in individual servings so you can grab them as you are running out the door.

- Make a point to include a vegetable with your lunch.

- Make sure to enjoy vegetables when you eat out at a restaurant or deli.

For a list of fruits and vegetables rich in soluble fiber, refer back to Step #1.

Step #8: MindLESS eating is the problem— MindFUL eating is the solution.

If Americans just ate more slowly, that would have a huge impact on our calorie intake and our mealtime enjoyment. What is MindLESS eating? Answer: when you are distracted and not fully paying attention while you eat. For example:

- You are so hungry that you almost inhale your food without noticing the flavors.

- Eating while concentrating on something else (TV, computer, driving, working).

- Following rules on what, when, and how much to eat (a diet).

- Eating past comfortable to miserably stuffed.

- Eating out of emotional rather than physical hunger.

- Eating directly from the box, bag, or carton.

- You finish a cookie and wish you had another bite because you weren't paying attention and truly tasting the cookie you just ate.

You make about 250 food decisions every day. Instead of indulging fear, anxiety, guilt, or obsession (these lead to more emotional eating, not less), approach food decisions with mindfulness! Mindful eating means choosing to eat food that is both pleasing to you and nourishing to your body while using all of your senses to explore, savor, and taste it. Mindful eating is vital to being healthy in mind, body, and spirit! Mindful eating is particularly helpful with foods high in enjoyment and low in nutritional value.

The four steps to mindful eating

#1: Understand physical feelings of hunger

- Eat when you are truly hungry and stop when you are comfortable.
- Physical hunger builds gradually whereas emotional hunger develops suddenly.
- Use a hunger scale to measure your hunger and fullness—just until you get better at judging your physical hunger and satisfaction/fullness.

#2: Slow eating equals satisfaction (big benefits from eating slowly)

- Connect with your body by taking a few deep breaths (it takes 20 minutes for your stomach to get the message to your brain that it is comfortably full).
- Take a moment to appreciate your food.

It just makes sense that the faster you eat your meal, the better the chance that you will consume more "extra" unnecessary calories. And the slower your eating rate, the more mindful you tend to be of the eating experience and the more time you are giving the stomach to tell the brain that it is now comfortable (and without hunger).

Recent research results demonstrated that if you want to eat fewer calories during your meal, you'd better slow down (*J Am Diet Assoc* [July 2008], 108(7): 1186–91). The 30 healthy women in the study reported:

- Satiety was significantly lower in the quick-eating group compared with the slow-eating group.
- People consumed less water in the fast-eating group compared with the slow-eating group (290 grams vs. 410 grams).
- People consumed more total calories in the fast-eating group compared with the slow-eating group (646 calories vs. 579 calories).

This difference in total meal calories (67 calories) might seem small at first, but over the course of a week, the calorie savings can add up. For example, a meal difference of 67 calories per meal, three times a day for seven days comes to about 1,400 calories a week. I can't help but think that for some people, a slower rate of eating might add up to even bigger weekly calorie savings.

Think about the times you've regrettably eaten way too much—way past eating comfortable and well on your way to a stuffed turkey. Were you super hungry for a while until you finally were able to get some food? Extreme hunger will inspire faster eating (or shoveling) and eating beyond comfortable in some people.

#3: Chew your food

- Chewing well aids digestion.
- Chewing allows you to engage the brain and enjoy the food flavors.
- The more you chew, the more likely you will be satisfied with less.
- Chewing enhances feelings of fullness.

#4: Engage all of your senses

To enjoy the food more fully, use taste, sight, aroma, and texture. Try this three-step exercise with food that is high in enjoyment but low in nutritional value:

1. Take a moment to connect with your body by taking a couple deep, centering breaths—appreciate the food and notice aromas, colors, and textures.
2. Place a small amount of the "high enjoyment" food in your mouth (the taste buds are on your tongue). Close your eyes and pay attention to the flavors and textures you are now experiencing. Let the chocolate or potato chip, for example, melt on its own at first.
3. Slowly begin to chew and eventually swallow when you are ready. The minute you swallow you stop tasting the food because the taste buds are on the tongue. Notice that when you take large bites, you tend to want to swallow quickly. When you take small bites, your mouth is more comfortable savoring and enjoying the morsel.

Note that when you enjoy and experience high-enjoyment food this way, even a Ghirardelli chocolate square (about four bites) or a fun-size Snickers (about six bites) is satisfying.

Make eating mindfully instead of mindlessly your priority!

Eating mindfully involves paying attention to hunger and satisfaction, being aware of and curious about why we are eating when we aren't hungry and learning from it. And mostly, eating mindfully means breathing deeply and being in gratitude before starting our meal, eating slowly, and allowing yourself to taste, savor, and find joy in every bite or sip.

Moderate "treats" with mindful eating tips
> Banning "treat" foods may eventually backfire by making those foods even more desirable. In research studies, girls who were allowed treats ate them moderately and tended to be thinner, whereas treat-deprived girls were found to eat larger amounts of banned foods when they weren't even hungry and tended to be thicker (*American Journal of Clinical Nutrition* [2003]; 78(2): 215–220).

Are humans designed to eat more?

Human beings have been able to survive food shortages in past centuries perhaps due, at least in part, to a genotype (genetic makeup) that permits, or even encourages, a calorie intake that is greater than the calories burned when food is abundant and available. This works really well when you are surviving the potato famine or a particularly harsh winter. But in modern times, with appetizing and affordable food absolutely everywhere, this can present a problem. The modern human can survive this food storm by staying as physically active as possible, by focusing on eating health-promoting foods most of the time, and, eating each meal in a relaxed and stress-free way. By eating slowly, we are at least giving ourselves the chance to enjoy the food and be more aware of our hunger being satisfied.

Not all calories are treated equally by the body

When it comes to promoting satiety (the sensation of having enough), of the three macronutrients (protein, carbohydrate, and fat), it's protein that wins the race, according to several studies. Second in line are carbohydrates and last is fat. Believe it or not, high fat foods were found to have a weak effect on satiety, even compared to sugar or sucrose. Think about how physically satisfying some of our favorite high-fat foods (not necessarily high in protein) are—foods like potato chips, french fries, and whipped cream. More than a decade ago, researchers measured the "satiety index" of common foods and found it was the more calorie dense, fat-rich foods that had the lower satiety index scores, and the bulky foods that were high in protein, fiber, or water that had the higher satiety scores.

When it comes to appetite and satiety, high-fat foods seem to present the perfect storm. Think about it—they are have more calories per gram weight than carbohydrates and protein (nine calories per gram compared to four), they tend to have high palatability (taste appeal), and they have been shown to have lower satiety values between meals and within the meal it's being consumed in. Given all of these matters at play, I'm not surprised that we tend to over-consume some of these high-fat foods.

More research needs to be done in this area, but keep in mind normal human satiety cues can be disrupted by other influences such as whether a person has dieted quite a bit (and practiced not eating when they are hungry), or whether they eat too much at times in an out of control way (bingeing).

10 tips to reduce emotional eating

Emotional eating may be in play if you reach for food because of the way you feel and not because you are physically hungry. If you think you are an emotional eater, know that you are not alone and that there are things you can do and professionals you can see who can help.

Knowing that you are vulnerable to emotional eating may be the first step, but learning how best to handle and curtail emotional eating episodes is probably the most challenging step. To help you with this, here are 10 tips to help you minimize emotional eating or food cravings.

Tip #1: Understanding real hunger vs. emotional eating

The first step to reducing emotional eating is understanding the difference between real hunger and emotional cravings. Real hunger occurs when your stomach feels physically empty. Has it been several hours since you've eaten your last meal or snack? There are different degrees of hunger too, from the slight feeling of an empty stomach to a more uncomfortable hunger and pain in the stomach. In research studies, Dr. Jean Kristeller, PhD, professor of psychology at Indiana State University and president of the board of directors at The Center for Mindful Eating, has used a number scale, with one being the lowest and 10 being the highest, to rate hunger and fullness. Megrette Fletcher, MEd, RD, CDE, cofounder of The Center for Mindful Eating, has found that the more often people use this number rating system, the better their ability to eat when comfortably hungry and stop when comfortably full. She also agrees that focusing on eating when you are hungry and stopping when you are comfortable is especially helpful when a person is eating for emotional reasons. Fletcher says: "Emotions that are strong can often distract us from physical cues like hunger and fullness, that in less stressful situations are used to regulate a person's intake" as said to me in an interview. She advises us to make a habit of asking these two questions (How hungry am I? How comfortable or full am I?) before, during, and toward the end of a meal.

It is easier to take the time to enjoy the food when you are eating in a slow and mindful way. The more you savor your food, the fewer bites you'll tend to need to satisfy your stomach and your emotions.

Tip #2: Don't skip meals

Eat a balanced diet with ample fiber and plant protein as they encourage stomach satisfaction. If you have a difficult schedule, pack along some healthy but convenient snacks so you can feed your physical hunger when it strikes and avoid moving into extreme hunger (which can make some people vulnerable to overeating).

Tip #3: Switch to healthful foods in general

Switch to more healthful foods when possible as part of your daily eating, and to satisfy some of your cravings—but wait until you are truly physically hungry to eat meals and snacks. I realize this may sound silly to some, but if you want to enjoy some ice cream, for example, there are great-tasting light ice-creams and frozen yogurts available. If it is fettuccine Alfredo you are yearning for, you can make a light and luscious Alfredo sauce and serve it over high fiber pasta for dinner that day. And serve it with lightly cooked broccoli too!

When you look at obesity research, the strongest evidence for an increased risk of obesity by eating a certain way is for diets that are high in dietary fat or low in fiber. It makes sense that eating an excess of foods high in fat might encourage extra fat on the body, and there are studies to support this way of thinking. Animal studies suggest that the body seems to prefer to store or deposit saturated fat, whereas unsaturated fats are more likely to be used or oxidized. And a large number of studies have shown that as fiber intake goes up, weight gain tends to go down. So moving yourself toward a healthier way of eating (high fiber, lower saturated fat) may also help you feel better about yourself and reduce the risk of obesity.

Researcher Brian Wansink, PhD, director of the Cornell Food and Brand Lab, asked more than a thousand Americans what their favorite comfort food is and why they indulge. Forty percent of the favorite comfort foods named were actually somewhat healthful or have the potential to be more healthful, such as pasta, pizza, soups, meats, and casseroles. And the news gets even better. Their research also found that people were more likely to seek out comfort foods when they were happy or when they wanted to reward themselves. A smaller percentage of the participants craved comfort foods when they were depressed or lonely (*Physiology and Behavior* [September 2003], 79(4–5), 739–747). I think this is good news because people are probably more likely to be in the frame of mind to switch to healthful choices and substitutions if they are in a happy mood rather than a sad one. People in sad moods, according to Dr. Wansink's research, tend to turn to sugary, fatty foods such as ice cream, cookies, or a bag of potato chips.

Tip #4: Uncover your true emotions

Uncover your true emotions within and get the professional help you need to fully deal with anything that is causing you pain, sadness, or anger. Many people tend to try to cover up their deepest emotions and find ways to escape or numb their pain. But all of these things are usually temporary fixes. Deep down, no matter how many adhesive bandages you find to cover it up, the underlying hurt or scar is still there.

Tip #5: Understand the roles of stress and boredom

When you aren't truly hungry but are craving food, ask yourself if you are bored or stressed. If so, discover ways of de-stressing or beating boredom without involving food. Studies suggest stress can encourage the act of eating, with a tendency toward sweet and fatty foods. A recent study showed that exposing rats to mild stress in the presence of food led to over-eating and obesity, whereas severe stress can do the opposite. Dr. Kristeller believes eating can become an automatic, unconscious response to tension and anxiety. "Learning to become more mindful in these moments can help you break that pattern of automatic reactivity," says Kristeller (interview with author, 2008). Dr. Kristeller suggests:

- Learning to recognize your stress signals.

- Enjoying what you are eating—how it tastes and smells and the various textures.

- Checking in with yourself and asking, *Do I really want to eat this? Is it going to be helpful?*

- Acknowledging your cravings. Create choices so *you* are in charge instead of the craving. Do you want to have one cookie now? Will that be better in the long run than trying to ignore it and having the urge become so overwhelming later that you eat half the bag?

- Evaluating your true hunger.

Tip #6: Changing emotional eating habits can be complicated

Everyone who has ever tried changing a long-term habit or behavior knows that it isn't easy. The most successful behavior modification programs have not only dispensed information but also helped shift motivation in their participants and provided the necessary skills to maintain the behavior change. See what I mean by "complicated"? Some of our emotional food cravings may even have a physiological explanation. New research from the University of Oxford revealed that several parts of the brain were more likely to respond to the sight and flavor of chocolate in people who habitually crave chocolate compared to non-chocolate cravers.

Tip #7: Is your eating environment helping or hurting?

Increasingly, research studies are acknowledging how hard it is to stay on the healthy eating track in modern society. Several factors exist in the typical eating environment today that can make it feel as though we are trying to swim upstream when we are trying to eat healthy and refrain from overeating or eating without physical hunger. Our current environment, for example, provides an abundance of tempting food, food variety, and food advertising.

All of these things make it even more difficult to eat when you are truly hungry and to stop when you are truly comfortable; they encourage overeating and eating out of emotion instead of physical hunger. Some research suggests that stress and pre-existing eating habits make it even more difficult to resist temptation.

Tip #8: Be aware of environmental eating cues

"There's a lot of merit in controlling the environmental cues like meal size, eating speed, and distractions," notes Megrette Fletcher.

Not only does it just make sense that certain cues encourage us to continue eating past the point of comfort, but research has supported this as well. When we are served a big meal or when we eat quickly or when we eat with distractions, we are usually not eating in a way that is mindful, slowly savoring the flavors. So, we are less likely to be aware of when our body is comfortable and satisfied so we can naturally stop eating. Studies have suggested that large portions of food tend to increase the calories we eat in a meal without an increase in satiety or satisfaction. And when people eat quickly, they aren't giving their body enough time to receive the signals of satiety.

Tip #9: Brush away evening emotions

Try the "clean your teeth" tip. After your last meal of the day, take some time to floss and brush your teeth. This sends a message to your subconscious that you are done eating for the night. Feel free to enjoy no-calorie liquids though! And if you are truly hungry, then by all means, consider eating a healthful, satisfying evening snack.

Tip #10: Be an avid water drinker!

Keep your hands, stomach, and mouth busy by drinking and enjoying all sorts of no-calorie beverages like water, hot or iced tea, sparkling water with lemon or lime, and even a cup or two of coffee (decaf if desired).

Avoid eating large meals

Eating more often, but smaller amounts at a time, is a good idea for some, but can be particularly helpful for some people with type 2 diabetes.

What small meals do for blood sugar levels

Small meals, spaced throughout the day (about every two-and-a-half to three hours) translate into more stable blood sugar throughout the day. Smaller meals generally result in smaller blood glucose responses, requiring less insulin and improving blood glucose control in some people with type 2 diabetes.

It makes sense that, often, the bigger the meal, the larger the number of calories eaten from carbohydrates, fat, and protein, and the higher the blood levels of those nutrients will be after the large meal. Large meals also zap you of your after-meal energy. If you've had a large meal, a nap is usually not far behind. But if you eat smaller meals, you will feel more energetic throughout your day. (Smaller, lower-fat meals don't stay in the stomach long; they move quickly to the intestines.) If you feel light on your feet, you are more likely to be physically active too. The more physically active, the more calories you will burn going about your day.

Other benefits of small meals

If you don't want to eat this way to help your diabetes, then do it for these other great reasons:

- Your brain and body require a constant supply of energy in the blood. Eating smaller, more frequent meals is more likely to keep your blood sugar (and energy) stable, preventing low blood sugar levels that can trigger headaches, irritability, food cravings, or overeating in susceptible people.

- Eating smaller meals more frequently is great for appetite control. The more stable blood sugar gained from smaller meals keep us from getting overly hungry, which can lead to overeating or making high-sugar or high-fat food choices.

- One study revealed that obesity was less common in people who ate more frequent meals. People who eat smaller, more frequent meals are less likely to overeat at any meal. Larger meals flood your bloodstream with a load of fat, protein, and carbohydrate calories, and your body has to get rid of any extra calories. What does this have to do with being overweight? All extra calories can be converted to body fat for energy storage.

- You burn more calories digesting, absorbing, and metabolizing your food just by eating more often. The body burns calories when it digests and absorbs the food we eat. And every time we eat, the digestion process goes into gear. If we eat six small meals instead of two large ones, we start the digestive process three times more often every single day, thereby burning more calories. This metabolism-inspired increase in calories burned can burn around five to 10 percent of the total calories we eat in a day.

- It's physically more comfortable to eat smaller meals. You aren't weighed down by a large meal in your stomach.

How frequent should the smaller meals be?

Experts have not yet determined the ideal eating pattern for people with diabetes, but so far it seems that the closer together the meals are, the better the results. The longer the gap between a previous meal or snack and dinner, for example, the larger the dinner typically ends up being.

If you eat a small breakfast, have a midmorning snack, a light lunch, then an afternoon snack, and a light dinner—it adds up to five small meals for the day. The best advice I can give you, until researchers know more, is to space your meals according to your individual schedule, when you tend to get hungry, and your blood glucose goals.

Fight the urge to eat at night

We burn 70 percent of our calories as fuel during the day, but when do many Americans eat the majority of their calories? During the evening hours. If we're eating small meals throughout the day, eating when we were hungry and stopping when we feel comfortable, it should be easier to avoid eating large dinners and evening desserts and snacks. Keep in mind that what you eat in the evening will be hitting your bloodstream pretty much around the time you are getting in your jammies. It isn't as though you are eating to fuel a marathon or anything.

Easier said than done

Our whole society is based on three meals a day, with dinner typically being the largest meal of the day. This is a hard habit to break. If you eat out often, it becomes particularly difficult not to eat a large meal. Restaurants tend to serve large meals—that's all there is to it. It requires extra diligence at restaurants to eat only half your meal and save the rest for later. If you are having spaghetti, you could eat the salad and half your entrée, and then have the garlic bread and the rest of your spaghetti later or the next day. I'm not saying it isn't going to be difficult, but it can be done.

A word of caution

Admittedly, for some people this way of eating four or five times a day may not be the best way; these are people who may have a difficult time stopping the eating process once they start. If this describes you, I invite you to visit The Center for Mindful Eating (*www.tcme.org*) for assorted resources to help you be more mindful every time you sit down to enjoy a mcal.

Step #9: Monitor your blood sugar.

Keeping your blood glucose as near to normal as possible protects your body from diabetic complications further down the line. Measuring your blood sugar levels on a fairly regular basis, then, is a necessary step toward tightly controlling them. Measuring your blood sugar will tell you whether you are meeting your treatment goals and whether the agreed-upon treatments (diet, exercise, or pharmacological) are working.

You are, hopefully, working with a dietitian or CTE who is helping you personalize your eating plan. Logging in your food, blood sugar, medications, and exercise every day shows your dietitian or diabetes educator how your blood sugar is being affected from day to day. They can then work with you on fine-tuning your diabetes care plan by adjusting medications, changing your desired number of carbohydrate grams, and encouraging activity at certain times.

About one-and-a-half hours after eating, you will know whether your blood sugar is within normal limits, high, or low. This is your greatest tool! Use it. Each of us reacts a little differently to each food, combination of foods, and amount of those foods. The only way you can learn your own personal reaction to a particular meal is to test your blood sugar one-and-a-half hours later. Once you begin testing and recording your blood sugar levels, you can look back to your records for clues as to why your readings were what they were. Look for clues in three areas:

1. Food and diet. (What foods and how much?)
2. A change in your exercise or activity schedule. (Did you exercise at your usual time for the usual duration?)
3. Medication. (Did you take the proper amount of medication at the proper time?)

Step #10: Make exercise fun, and do it every day!

When you exercise regularly, you just plain feel better. You burn more calories, and you increase your muscle mass, which increases your metabolic rate. And that's just the beginning. Exercising will help decrease blood sugar levels and, possibly, the dose of insulin you need to take. It will decrease blood cholesterol levels and bone loss while improving your circulation, heart function, and your ability to deal with stress. Obviously, exercise has huge health pay-offs. Make exercise a priority and a habit, please!

Four reasons why many people don't exercise

1. It isn't fun! It isn't exercise per se that isn't fun; it's the *type* of exercise that you have been doing that you are not finding fun. Think about all the possible types of exercise and write down which ones you might find the most enjoyable.

Also, think about what types of exercise you don't like and try to put your finger on why they're not fun. This will give you some clues about what your fun exercise options might be.

If you dislike the types of exercise that you do alone, then perhaps you would like exercise that is done as group or team. If you don't think exercising at home is fun, then you should think about exercises that are—water aerobics, walking with a buddy, country western dance lessons, and so on—that you can do somewhere close to your home.

2. There's just no time! We make time for the things we really *want* to do, don't we? And we make time for the things we really *have* to do too. If exercising makes us feel better (and we make it fun), then hopefully it will become something we really *want* to do. If exercising helps us control our blood sugar and body weight (and it does!), then it is also something we really *have* to do for our health.

Keep in mind that fitting even 10 minutes of exercise here and there, during our day, can help your body manage diabetes. Walking after a meal or snack (or during a time when your blood sugar tends to be too high) can be particularly helpful for diabetics. The exercise helps move and use the blood sugar in your bloodstream. This doesn't have to be jogging or swimming right after a meal, it could be a quick, 10-minute jaunt around your office building after lunch, taking the stairs, or walking the dog after dinner.

3. It's boring! You may be someone who needs to plan variety into your exercise program. You might want to join a class (dance, jazzercise, water aerobics, swimming, golf, basketball, or tennis) that meets two or three days a week, then fill in the other days with walks, weight training, cycling, and so on. Take lessons for a sport you actually find interesting.

For many of us, exercising at home on a machine is most convenient. If you work out for 30 minutes, then it takes exactly 30 minutes out of your day. I ride my stationary bike while I watch a television movie or program that I'm dying to see. I even fast forward through the commercials if I'm watching a tape. The television keeps my interest as my body is doing the work. You may want to listen to some of your favorite CDs or maybe even an audio book.

4. It's raining, it's pouring! Having several types of exercise options available to you not only adds variety (and minimizes boredom), but it gives you an automatic bad weather plan. If you have home exercise equipment, use it when the weather is cold or wet. If you have signed up for exercise classes or sports leagues, they are usually indoors, so you know you will at least get some exercise on those days each week.

If you like to walk and you have a walking buddy depending on you, you could very well decide to walk rain or shine. As long as it isn't raining too hard, my walking buddy and I just put on our hooded ski jackets and brave the drops. I find it invigorating! And the warm shower afterwards is truly therapeutic.

Chapter 5

The Recipes You Can't Live Without

This chapter is designed to give you just a sampling of possible recipes to start you on the road to more healthful cooking. Some of the recipes are from scratch, whereas others make use of the countless convenient products now available. Hopefully you will find a handful that suit you and your family perfectly. For more recipes, check out my Website: *www.recipedoctor.com*. I also have a cookbook that might come in handy: *Food Synergy* (Rodale, March 2008).

Most of us cook the same recipes over and over again, so I wanted to give you some recipe guidelines to lighten up your own family favorites!

Smart substitutions

Healthy food isn't going to do anyone any good if no one is eating it. That's been my motto for the 25 years that I've been "lightening" recipes. In other words, even if it's light, it's gotta taste right.

Lightening recipes comes down to basically three things: trimming extra saturated fat and switching to smart fats when possible, trimming extra sugar and sugar-containing ingredients, and switching to whole grains and adding fiber-rich foods when possible.

The specific keys to successful lightening are:

- Find the ideal fat and sugar threshold for the recipe. How much can you cut calories, saturated fat, and sugar without compromising flavor and texture? See the following table for more help on this.

- Use the fat substitute that works best in that recipe. See the table for more help on this also.

- Review the functions of each fatty or sweet ingredient before you make changes to your recipe. When fat or sugar serves an irreplaceable function, you'll probably need to keep some of it in, but you can usually cut fat in half and sugar by one-third.

- Substitute reduced-fat and reduced-sugar ingredients and products when appropriate. For example, use reduced-fat sharp cheddar instead of regular, use a good-tasting fat-free or light sour cream instead of regular, or use fat-free half-and-half or low-fat milk instead of cream. You can also use reduced-calorie pancake syrup, unsweetened frozen fruit, and so on, instead of regular.

- When possible, change to a cooking method that eliminates the need for cooking fat (such as broiling, roasting, poaching, and steaming). But when cooking fat is necessary to maintain the character of the food, just use less of it for your oven frying, browning, or sautéing or pan frying, and switch to a smart fat whenever possible (such as canola oil or extra virgin olive oil).

Ideal fat thresholds and substitutions

Based on two decades of experimentation with the best ways to lighten recipes, I've discovered that there are ideal fat thresholds that you must keep for flavor and texture. If you cut back the fat in a particular recipe, you'll need a fat replacement an extra ingredient you can add to help replace the fat and moisture you have taken out.

For example, if you are making brownies and you cut the butter back from eight tablespoons to three, you can add five tablespoons of fat-free sour cream to the batter to make up the difference. You can also use half whole-wheat flour to increase the fiber and you can often reduce the sugar by a third or fourth.

If you are making a spice cake using a cake mix, don't add the half cup of oil the recipe requires; add half a cup of unsweetened applesauce (or some other fat replacement) instead.

Recipe	Fat Threshold	Fat Replacements
Biscuits/scones	4 Tbs. shortening for every 2 cups flour.	Fat-free cream cheese, nonfat or light sour cream, flavored yogurt.
Cake mixes	No additional fat is needed because most mixes already contain fat in the mix.	Instead of adding the oil called for on the box, add applesauce, liqueur, fruit juice, flavored yogurt, or nonfat sour cream, depending on the cake.
Brownies	2 1/2 Tbs. canola oil or butter per 4 oz. unsweetened chocolate and about 14 Tbs. flour.	Fat-free sour cream works well, along with espresso or strong coffee.
Homemade cakes and coffee cakes	1/4 to 1/3 cup fat ingredient per cake.	Liqueur for some cakes, light sour cream for chocolate ones; fruit purees and juices work well with carrot, apple, and spice cakes.
Cheese sauce	No butter is needed, so omit the butter if it is called for. The cheese is the vital fatty ingredient; use a reduced-fat cheddar.	Make your thickening paste by mixing the flour with a little bit of milk, then whisk in the remaining milk called for in the recipe.
Cookies	Generally you can only cut the fat by half. If the original recipe calls for 1 cup of butter, try cutting it to 1/2 cup.	Fat-free cream cheese for rich cookies; some fruit purees may work in fruit/drop cookies.

Marinades	1 Tbs. oil per cup of marinade (or none at all).	Fruit juices or beer help to balance the sharpness of the more acid ingredients in a marinade such as vinegar or tomato juice.
Muffins and nut bread	2 Tbs. oil for a 12-muffin recipe.	Fat-free sour cream, low-fat flavored yogurts, fruit juice, and fruit purees.
Vinagrette dressings	1 to 2 Tbs. olive oil per 1/2 cup dressing.	Wine or champagne, fruit juice, fruit purees (raspberry and pear work well).
Cake mixes	1 tsp. butter per serving of sauce	Add a little more milk. I like to use whole milk or fat-free half and half for a rich white sauce.

Here are a few more substitution or fat-reduction tips to use when cooking various dishes:

- In mostly egg dishes, you can cut the eggs in half and replace the lost eggs with Egg Beaters egg substitute (1/4 cup substitute per egg).

- Many recipes call for using much more oil or butter in pan frying or sautéing than is really necessary. Using a teaspoon of olive or canola oil at the most, per serving, usually does the trick with non-stick pans.

- If you can switch to canola or olive oil instead of using solid fat or shortening in a recipe, do it! These oils contain healthier fats (monounsaturated fat and canola oil also contains omega-3s) than the saturated fats in shortening, butter, and stick margarines.

Living well with diabetes: a sample menu

Most people with diabetes have learned that what you choose to eat and drink can help raise or lower your blood sugar levels after meals. There are basically four components in food that can affect your blood sugar—carbohydrates, fiber, protein, and fat. Though fiber, protein and, to a lesser extent, fat, can blunt the blood sugar rise after a meal, it's mostly carbohydrates that can raise blood sugar, and mostly fat that can increase insulin resistance.

Aiming for a balance of carbohydrates, protein, and fat in your meals can be helpful to many people with diabetes, but a crucial next step is to emphasize quality carbohydrates and smart fats: vegetables, beans, whole grains, and fruit for carbohydrates; and fish, nuts and seeds, avocado, olives, extra virgin olive oil, and canola oil for fat.

Everybody with diabetes will respond a little differently to the same meal, so checking your blood sugar regularly (two hours after a meal), and looking for patterns between what you eat and drink and the blood sugar levels that result, will help you take charge of your diabetes.

The sample menus and recipes that follow include meals that are balanced with carbohydrates, protein, fat, and a great source of fiber, and emphasize the foods that are sources of quality carbohydrates and smart fats suggested previously.

Sample daily menu

Breakfast

High fiber carbohydrate food (choose from the following):
- Whole-grain cereals (hot or cold).
- Whole-grain bread, English muffin, or bagel (for French toast or on the side).
- Whole-grain waffles/pancakes.
- Vegetables such as spinach, broccoli, tomatoes—if egg-based breakfast entrée.
- Fresh or frozen fruit (add to cereal, smoothie, yogurt, or pancakes/waffles).

Lean protein food/drink (low in saturated fat):
- Higher omega-3 egg blended with two egg whites for egg dish.
- Low-fat milk or soymilk for hot or cold cereal or as beverage.
- Part-skim cheese (for toast or egg dishes).
- Low- or nonfat yogurt (ingredient in smoothie or enjoy with cereal).

Possible smart fats:
- Avocado for egg dishes.
- Nuts for cereals and yogurt parfait.
- Extra virgin olive oil used in egg dishes.
- Canola oil used in whole-grain muffins, pancakes, and waffles.

Lunch

Sandwich or wrap made with whole-grain bread or tortilla and a lean protein such as:

- Roasted turkey or chicken (skinless) or lean beef or pork.
- Part-skim cheese or soy cheese.
- Tuna—water packed—dressed in a vinaigrette or yogurt instead of mayo.
- Falafels or other bean- or soy-based filling.
- Roasted vegetables.

Bean-based lunch such as:
- Bean burrito.
- Hummus with whole-grain bread or veggie dippers.
- Chili (with lean meat or vegetarian version) or stew featuring beans.

Entrée salad made with dark green lettuce, plenty of vegetables, lean meat or fish, or beans, or cheese plus avocado and nuts, if desired. Dressing made with extra virgin olive oil or canola oil or yogurt.

Dinner

High-fiber carbohydrate (choose from the following):
- Cooked grains like brown rice, quinoa, barley, bulgur, amaranth, etc.
- Whole wheat breads (tortilla, pita, buns, etc.).
- Colorful vegetables on the side or with the entrée.
- Dark green lettuce for side or dinner salad.
- Fresh fruit on the side or with the entrée.

Lean protein food (low in saturated fat):
- Grilled or baked fish (by itself or in a mixed dish such as tacos).
- Skinless poultry (grilled, baked, or stir-fried).
- Lean beef or pork (sirloin, tenderloin) with no visible fat.
- Part-skim cheese in entrees (macaroni and cheese, eggplant parmesan, vegetarian pizza on whole wheat crust, vegetable lasagna, enchiladas, etc.).

Possible smart fats:
- Extra virgin olive oil or canola used in sensible amounts to cook the previous dishes.
- Nuts as an ingredient for entrée or side dishes.
- Avocado or olives with entrée or side dishes.

Now let's get cooking! Here are some recipes to get you started on your way!

Three ground flax recipes

Honey-Wheat Rolls
Makes 16 dinner rolls.

    1/4 cup concentrated decaf coffee (espresso-strength).
1 1/4 cups warm water.
2 Tbs. canola oil.
1/3 cup honey.
1 1/2 cups unbleached white flour.
1/2 cup ground flaxseed.
1 3/4 cups whole-wheat flour.
1 1/2 Tbs. unsweetened cocoa.
1 tsp. salt.
1 package bread machine yeast (about 2 1/4 tsp.).
Canola oil cooking spray.

1. Add all ingredients except yeast and cooking spray to your bread machine in the order listed. Once everything has been added, make a well in the center of the flour and pour in the yeast.
2. Set the machine on the dough cycle (this normally takes around one hour and 40 minutes). When the timer goes off, shape the dough into 16 dinner rolls and let them rise on baking sheets coated with cooking spray.
3. Let the rolls rise until they double in size (about 45 minutes). Preheat oven to 350 degrees. Bake until cooked throughout and browned on the outside (about 15 to 20 minutes). Enjoy the rolls while they are still warm!

Per roll: 147 calories, 4 g protein, 25 g carbohydrate, 3.5 g fat, 0.2 g saturated fat, 0 mg cholesterol, 4 g fiber, 146 mg sodium. Calories from fat: 21 percent. 1.2 g omega-3 fatty acids.

Flaxseed Jam Muffins
Makes nine regular sized muffins.

 Canola cooking spray.
1/8 cup nonfat or light sour cream.
1/8 cup canola oil.
1/2 cup low-fat milk.

1/4 cup egg substitute (or 1 egg).

2 Tbs. light corn syrup.

1 tsp. vanilla extract.

2/3 cup unbleached flour.

2/3 cup whole-wheat flour.

1/3 cup ground flaxseed.

1/2 cup granulated sugar.

2 tsp. baking powder.

1/2 tsp. salt.

4 Tbs. reduced-sugar jam of your choice.

1. Preheat oven to 375 degrees. Coat nine muffin cups with canola cooking spray.

2. Place sour cream in a glass mixing bowl and warm briefly in the microwave so it will blend more easily. Stir in oil and milk, a tablespoon at a time. Stir in egg or egg substitute, corn syrup, and vanilla extract.

3. Blend dry ingredients together (flours, flaxseed, sugar, baking powder, salt) and add all at once to liquid mixture. Stir just enough to moisten.

4. Fill each muffin cup with a level 1/4 cup measure of batter. Spoon about 1 1/2 teaspoons of jam in the center of each muffin. Bake about 18 to 20 minutes or until golden brown and muffin tests done.

Per serving (using reduced-sugar jam): 197 calories, 4.5 g protein, 35.5 g carbohydrate, 5 g fat, 0.5 g saturated fat, 1 mg cholesterol, 3 g fiber, 260 mg sodium. Calories from fat: 23 percent. Omega-3 fatty acids: 1.5 g.

Flaxseed Maple Scones

If you even barely like the taste of maple, you will find these scones addicting! I even adjusted the recipe for a food processor to make these scones a cinch to make. These scones are loaded with ground flaxseed, so one scone will give you a day's supply of flaxseed. They freeze well in plastic resealable bags. You can even eat them right out of the freezer!

Makes eight scones.

Scones:

1 1/2 cups all-purpose flour.

1/3 cup oats.

1/2 cup ground flaxseed.

2 Tbs. sugar.

1/2 tsp. salt.

1 Tbs. baking powder.

2 Tbs. maple syrup.

2 Tbs. canola oil.

1 egg.

1/2 cup whole milk (low-fat milk will work too).

1/2 tsp. maple extract (3/4 tsp. if you prefer a stronger maple flavor).

2/3 cup pecans, coarsely chopped (a little smaller than "pecan pieces" but bigger than "finely chopped" pecans).

Canola cooking spray.

Maple Glaze:

1 1/2 cups powdered sugar.

1/2 tsp. maple extract.

5 tsp. water.

1. Preheat oven to 425 degrees. Make an 8-inch circle with canola cooking spray on a thick baking sheet.
2. Add flour, oats, flaxseed, sugar, salt, and baking powder to the food processor bowl. Pulse to mix and finely grind the oats with the flour.
3. Add maple syrup and canola oil to the flour mixture and pulse to blend well.
4. In a separate small bowl, beat the egg lightly with the milk and 1/2 tsp. maple extract. Pour the milk mixture into the flour mixture in the food processor. Pulse briefly to make a dough.
5. Place dough on a well-floured surface. Sprinkle pecans over the top and knead lightly four times to evenly distribute the pecans. Pat the dough into a 7 1/2-inch circle. Cut it into eight wedges. Place the wedges in a circle on a prepared baking sheet. Bake them in the center of the oven for about 13–15 minutes (the tops will be lightly browned).
6. While the scones are baking, add glaze ingredients to a small bowl and stir well until smooth. Remove the scones from the oven to the wire rack and let cool about three to five minutes. Spread the glaze generously over each scone. Once the glaze has dried (about 15 minutes) the scones can be served! They keep well overnight in a resealable plastic bag.

Per serving: 330 calories, 6 g protein, 51 g carbohydrate, 12 g fat, 4 g fiber, 38 mg cholesterol, 370 mg sodium. Calories from fat: 33 percent. Omega-3 fatty acids: 1.3 g.

Note: Because the fat grams mainly come from the pecans and the canola oil, most of the fat is the preferred monounsaturated fat!

Six recipes featuring intact whole grains

Quinoa and Edamame Salad (Vegan)

Makes about nine servings (1/2 cup each).

Ingredients:

3 cups cooked quinoa (1 cup dry); quinoa can be cooked in a rice cooker, just like rice.

1 cup edamame from frozen (shelled); micro-cook on high until tender (asparagus pieces can also be used).

1/3 cup dried cranberries.

1/2 cup sunflower seeds or walnut pieces, roasted or toasted.

Garden Vinaigrette:

1 Tbs. Dijon mustard.

1 Tbs. finely chopped shallot or 2 tablespoons chopped green onions.

2 Tbs. cider vinegar.

1/4 tsp. salt.

1/4 tsp. white pepper.

1/4 cup extra virgin olive oil.

2 tsp. fresh sage, chopped (1/2 tsp. dried).

2 tsp. fresh oregano, chopped (1/2 tsp. dried).

2 tsp. fresh thyme, chopped (1/2 tsp. dried).

Directions:

1. Combine the first four ingredients in a serving bowl and mix well.
2. Add the first six vinaigrette ingredients to a mini food processor and pulse to blend into an emulsion. Add the herbs and adjust the salt and pepper to taste (if desired).
3. If you don't have a mini food processor (or similar), whisk the first five vinaigrette ingredients together in a medium bowl. Slowly drizzle in the olive oil, whisking constantly to form an emulsion. Add herbs and adjust the salt and pepper to taste (if desired).
4. Keep refrigerated until ready to serve!

Per serving: 190 calories, 5 g protein, 16 g carbohydrate, 10 g fat, 1.2 g saturated fat, 5 g monounsaturated fat, 3.7 g polyunsaturated fat, 0 mg cholesterol, 3 g fiber, 110 mg sodium. Omega-3 fatty acids: 0.7 g. Omega-6 fatty acids: 3 g.

Black Bean Quinoa Salad With Avocado-Lime Dressing

Makes four servings.

1 (15 oz.) can of black beans, rinsed and drained.

3/4 cup dry quinoa, cooked in a rice cooker (approx. 2 1/4 cup cooked).

1/4 cup finely chopped red onion (sweet onion can be substituted).

1 cup cherry or grape tomatoes, cut in half.

Avocado-Lime Dressing:

1 small avocado or 1/2 large avocado, pitted, peeled, and chopped.

2 Tbs. lime juice.

1 Tbs. extra virgin olive oil.

1/4 cup fresh chopped cilantro (parsley can be substituted if desired).

Salt to taste (optional).

1. In a serving bowl, toss the beans, quinoa, red onion and tomatoes together.
2. Add the avocado-lime dressing ingredients to a mini food processor or blender and blend until smooth. Drizzle over the salad ingredients and stir to blend everything. Cover and chill until served.

Per serving: 235 calories, 8 g protein, 34 g carbohydrate, 7.5 g fat, 1 g saturated fat, 5 g monounsaturated fat, 1.5 g polyunsaturated fat, 0 mg cholesterol, 8 g fiber, 266 mg sodium. Calories from fat: 28 percent. Omega-3 fatty acids: 0.2 g. Omega-6 fatty acids: 1.3 g.

Kale Kamut Berry Salad
Makes six servings.

5 cups kale, shredded or chopped into thin strips.

1 1/4 cup cooked kamut (other intact whole grain can be substituted such as barley or wheat berries).

1 cup blueberries.

2 cups sliced strawberries.

1/3 to 1/2 cup reduced-fat crumbled feta cheese (optional).

6–8 Tbs. lite raspberry walnut vinaigrette (bottled, such as Ken's Steak House).

1/2 cup toasted pecans halves or walnut pieces (toast nuts in nonstick pan over medium heat, stirring often until fragrant and golden brown).

1. Add all the ingredients except nuts to a large salad serving bowl and toss to blend.
2. Sprinkle the nuts over the top and serve!

Per serving: 194 calories, 6 g protein, 28.5 g carbohydrates, 6.5 g fat, 0.9 g saturated fat, 1.5 g monounsaturated fat, 4 g polyunsaturated fat, 0 mg cholesterol, 3.5 g fiber, 150 mg sodium. Calories from fat: 30 percent. Omega-3 fatty acids: 1.4 g. Omega-6 fatty acids: 2.6 g.

Buckwheat Blender Crepes

Add the cinnamon and vanilla if you are making fruit filled or dessert crepes and if making an entrée crepe, add the suggested herbs instead of the cinnamon.

Makes seven crepes.

2/3 cup buckwheat groats (roasted or unroasted).

1 1/3 cups water.

1/2 cup low-fat milk.

1 Tbs. canola oil.

1 large egg, higher omega-3 if available.

2 Tbs. light pancake syrup.

1/4 tsp. ground cinnamon (replace with a Tbs. of chopped chives or green onion—or 1/2 tsp. of dried herb of your choice—if making a savory crepe).

1/4 tsp. salt.

1 tsp. vanilla extract (optional).

1. Add buckwheat groats in 2 cup measure or similar. Add 1 1/3 cups hot water and let sit overnight (minimum of four hours). Drain and rinse the groats well and then drain again.
2. Add all the ingredients into the blender and blend on increasing speed until the batter is smooth.
3. Preheat nonstick skillet on medium-high heat. Pour 1/4 cup of batter into the skillet. Tilt the skillet around to form a circle with crepe batter. Cook until the bottom is golden brown, about a minute, then flip to the other side to lightly brown. Remove from the skillet and repeat with remaining batter.
4. Fill crepes with fresh fruit for a breakfast or dessert crepe, or with chicken or shrimp salad (or similar) for an entrée crepe.

Per serving: 98 calories, 3.3 g protein, 14 g carbohydrate, 3 g fat, 0.7 g saturated fat, 1.5 g monounsaturated fat, 0.7 g polyunsaturated fat, 32 mg cholesterol, 2 g fiber, 114 mg sodium. Calories from fat: 29 percent. Omega-3 fatty acids: 0.2 g. Omega-6 fatty acids: 0.5 g.

Crock-pot Coconut Curry Chicken Casserole

If you choose, you can use light coconut milk instead of fat free half and half and coconut extract. You get your vegetables, whole grains, and lean meat all in one delicious dish. While the chicken is browning on the skillet, you can be adding the rest of the ingredients to the slow cooker, and everything cooks, including the dry brown rice, over the next four to six hours.

Makes four servings.
1 Tbs. extra virgin olive oil (or canola oil).
4 skinless, boneless chicken breasts.
Ground pepper.
Salt to taste (optional).
2 cups fat-free half and half.
2 tsp. coconut extract.
2 cups reduced-sodium chicken broth.
1 1/2 to 2 tsp. red curry powder.
3/4 cup uncooked brown rice (or other similar intact whole grain like barley, quinoa, or wheat berries).
2 small, red bell peppers (ribs and seeds removed), cut into thin strips or 1-inch pieces.
3 cups fresh or frozen green beans (stem ends removed), cut into 1-inch long pieces.
Garnish: 2 Tbs. toasted coconut, natural unsweetened or flaked (optional).

1. Begin heating the olive oil in a large nonstick skillet or frying pan over medium-high heat. Season the chicken with pepper and salt (if desired) and place it in the skillet to brown well on both sides (about three minutes a side).
2. While the chicken is browning, in a slow cooker dish combine fat-free half and half, coconut extract, chicken broth, red curry, and brown rice. Add the browned chicken on top and arrange the bell pepper and green beans over the top of the chicken. Cover the slow cooker and heat on low for four to six hours (or until the rice or other whole grain is tender).
3. Serve the chicken with some of the rice, vegetables, and curry coconut sauce and sprinkle some toasted coconut over the chicken if desired. Toast the coconut on a stove by spreading the shredded coconut in the bottom of a nonstick skillet or frying pan and cook over medium heat, stirring frequently, until the coconut is golden brown.

Per serving: 371 calories, 36 g protein, 40 g carbohydrate, 7.5 g fat, 1.7 g saturated fat, 4 g monounsaturated fat, 1.4 g polyunsaturated fat, 75 mg cholesterol, 5.5 g fiber, 271 mg sodium. Calories from fat: 18 percent. Omega-3 fatty acids: 0.1 g. Omega-6 fatty acids: 1.3 g.

 # High Legume Fried Rice
Makes four servings.

3 Tbs. canola oil.
1/4 cup green onions, sliced, firmly packed.
3/4 cup frozen green peas.

3/4 cup shelled edamame (if using frozen pods, follow the directions on the bag to finish cooking, and then remove the soy beans from the pods before measuring).

1/2 cup diced lean ham (optional).

4 cups cooked steamed brown rice.

1 egg beaten with 1/4 cup egg substitute.

1/2 tsp. salt.

1 to 2 Tbs. light or regular soy sauce.

1. Heat the oil in a wok or large nonstick saucepan to very hot. Add green onion and let sit for one minute.
2. Add green peas, soy beans, ham, and rice. Let stand for a minute.
3. Push away the mixture toward the edges of the pan, leaving the middle of the pan open, and pour in the egg mixture.
4. Let sit for about 20 seconds, and then begin to stir the eggs for another 20 seconds.
5. Stir fry the entire mixture together for a couple of minutes, sprinkling salt and soy sauce over the top. Add more soy sauce at table if desired.

Per serving: (with 2 Tbs. light soy sauce) 412 calories, 14.5 g protein, 64 g carbohydrate, 10 g fat, 1.5 g saturated fat, 53 mg cholesterol, 9 g fiber, 590 mg sodium. Calories from fat: 28 percent.

Six recipes featuring beans and legumes

Stove Top Fish Tacos with Mango Avocado Black Bean Salsa

This recipe works well with frozen fish. Just thaw fish in the refrigerator overnight.

Makes four servings.

Marinade:

2 Tbs. extra virgin olive oil.

2 Tbs. lime juice.

3/4 teaspoon chili powder.

3/4 tsp. dried oregano flakes.

1/4 tsp. ground cumin.

2 Tbs. lightly packed fresh cilantro leaves, finely chopped.

1/2 jalapeno, stemmed, and finely chopped (optional).

Fish: 1 pound flaky white fish (cod, tilapia, etc.) cut in about 4 pieces.

Mango Avocado Salsa:

2 Tbs. lightly packed fresh cilantro leaves, finely chopped.
2 Tbs. finely chopped red onion.
1 Tbs. lime juice.
1 Tbs. extra virgin olive oil.
1/2 avocado, pitted and finely diced.
1/2 mango, finely diced.
1/2 cup canned black beans (lower sodium), drained and rinsed.
2 cups finely shredded red, green, or Napa cabbage.
8 higher fiber corn tortillas.

1. Combine the marinade ingredients in a medium bowl. Place the fish pieces in the bowl and cover them well with marinade. Marinate for 20 minutes.
2. While the fish is marinating, combine the mango avocado salsa ingredients in a small serving bowl; set aside. Shred the cabbage if you haven't already and place in the medium serving bowl.
3. To heat and soften corn tortillas using your microwave: place four tortillas at a time on a plate between two lightly damp paper towels and microwave on high for about 30 seconds.
4. To heat and soften corn tortillas using the stove: begin heating a large, nonstick frying pan over medium-high heat. Coat both sides of the tortilla lightly with canola or olive oil cooking spray and lightly brown in a pan, flipping the tortilla to soften and lightly brown both sides. Repeat for the remaining tortillas.
5. To cook the fish, heat the large, nonstick frying pan over medium-high heat until good and hot. Add the fish pieces along with all of the marinade; season the fish lightly with freshly ground salt if desired. Cover the frying pan and reduce heat to low and cook the fish for four minutes undisturbed. Turn the fish over, cover the frying pan, and cook for four minutes more. Remove the pan from heat and let it cool for a couple of minutes in pan. Flake the fish in the pan with a fork and stir to blend with the juices left in the pan.
6. Everyone can make their own tacos, adding the cabbage to the tortillas, then the fish, and then the salsa!

Per serving: 352 calories, 23 g protein, 35 g carbohydrate, 14 g fat, 2 g saturated fat, 10 g monounsaturated fat, 2 g polyunsaturated fat, 43 mg cholesterol, 10 g fiber, 151 mg sodium. Calories from fat: 35 percent. Omega-3 fatty acids: 0.4 g. Omega-6 fatty acids: 1.6 g.

Texas Tater Skins

Makes 10 potato skins.

5 medium-sized russet potatoes (or red or white potato as well).

1 cup canned beans with a BBQ flavor (such as Bush's Grillin' Beans Texas Ranchero or Southern Pit BBQ).

1 cup shredded reduced-fat or regular cheese of choice (such as shredded reduced-fat sharp cheddar with reduced-fat Jack cheese).

1/3 cup chopped green onions (white and part green).

10 Tbs. fat-free or light sour cream (optional).

1. Pierce each potato a couple of times with a fork and microwave (following your microwave instructions for baked potatoes) until tender.
2. Let potatoes cool slightly then cut in half lengthwise and scoop out some of the center of each half, leaving plenty of potato with the skin. Place the skins on a cookie sheet or jellyroll pan.
3. Spoon a heaping tablespoon of canned beans down the center of each half. Top each half with shredded cheese of your choice and green onions if desired. Broil about six inches from the heat until the cheese is bubbling, then top with green onions (if you haven't already) and add a dollop of fat-free or light sour cream to each skin if desired. Serve to your hungry, football-lovin' crowd!

Per potato skin: 92 calories, 5 g protein, 11 g carbohydrate, 3 g fat, 1.9 g saturated fat, 0.5 g monounsaturated fat, 0.5 g polyunsaturated fat, 9 mg cholesterol, 2 g fiber, 202 mg sodium. Calories from fat: 29 percent.

Edamame With Buckwheat Soba Salad

If you have a bottled Thai peanut sauce that you like (such as Annie Chun's Gluten Free Thai Peanut Dipping Sauce), just add about six tablespoons to the noodles instead of making the peanut soy dressing from scratch.

Makes four servings.

3.1 ounces dry buckwheat soba noodles, cooked, and drained (follow directions on bag) Note: Available at Whole Foods markets and possibly the Asian section of your supermarket.

Peanut Soy Dressing:

3 Tbs. natural style peanut butter.

2 Tbs. of the noodle water.

4 1/2 tsp. soy sauce.

1 tsp. sesame oil.

2/3 cup shelled edamame, microwave for a few minutes to cook till tender.

Grilled protein of your choice, cut into bite-size pieces (1 cup if skinless chicken breast or lean beef, and 1 1/2 cups if extra-firm tofu* or tempch).

2–4 Tbs. chopped green onions (optional).

1. Add cooked and drained noodles to a serving bowl. In a mini food processor or similar, combine peanut soy dressing ingredients until desired consistency. To thin, just add more of the noodle water.

2. Drizzle peanut sauce over noodles and gently stir in the tender edamame, tofu, or grilled chicken and green onions if desired. Serve as a main dish or side salad.

* To grill the tofu, cut a block of tofu into about 1/3-inch wide slices. Marinate in balsamic or Asian dressing vinaigrette and grill on an indoor or outdoor grill. You can also buy tofu and tempeh already marinated and cooked in most supermarkets.

Per serving: 269 calories, 16 g protein, 23 g carbohydrate, 13 g fat, 1.4 g saturated fat, 0 mg cholesterol, 4 g fiber, 413 mg sodium. Calories from fat: 37 percent. Omega-3 fatty acids: 0.4 g.

Easy and Light Huevos Rancheros
Makes two servings.

2 whole-wheat or multigrain flour tortillas.

Canola oil or cooking spray.

2 large eggs blended with 1/2 egg substitute (or 1 cup egg substitute instead if desired).

Black pepper to taste.

1/3 cup shredded reduced-fat Jack or cheddar cheese.

1/2 cup canned black beans, rinsed and drained.

3 Tbs. bottled salsa (use your favorite).

2 heaping Tbs. fat-free sour cream.

1/2 small avocado, sliced.

1/2 vine-ripened medium tomato, chopped.

1. Begin heating a medium nonstick skillet over medium-high heat. Lay a tortilla in the skillet and flip over when underside is lightly brown. Lightly brown the other side of the tortilla and set aside. Repeat with the remaining tortilla.

2.   Reduce heat to medium-low and brush the bottom of the skillet lightly with canola oil using a silicon brush or coat with canola cooking spray. Pour in egg substitute or egg mixture and cook, stirring frequently, until the eggs are cooked to your desired texture (about two minutes). Turn off heat and add black pepper to taste. Sprinkle cheese over the top of the eggs and cover skillet.

3.   While the cheese is melting, combine black beans with salsa in a small bowl.

4.   To assemble huevos rancheros, top each of the crisp tortillas with half of the scrambled egg mixture, half of the black bean mixture, a dollop of sour cream, and half of the avocado slices and chopped tomato.

Per serving: 398 g calories, 40 g carbohydrate, 26 g protein, 15 g fat, 4 g saturated fat, 220 mg cholesterol (if 2 eggs were used), 12 g fiber, 775 mg sodium. Calories from fat: 33 percent.

The 3-Minute Burrito

Makes one burrito.

1/2 cup cooked or canned pinto beans or pinquitos (small brown beans), drained and rinsed.

1 Tbs. chopped fresh cilantro (optional).

2 Tbs. light or fat-free sour cream.

1 green onion, chopped.

1/8 cup chunky salsa (mild or hot, depending on preference).

1 burrito-size whole-wheat or whole-grain flour tortilla.

1 1/2 ounces reduced-fat Monterey jack or sharp cheddar cheese, grated (about a heaping 1/3 cup).

1.   In a small bowl, toss beans, cilantro, sour cream, green onion, and salsa together.

2.   Heat the tortilla in a microwave on a double thickness of paper towel for about one minute or until soft.

3.   Sprinkle the cheese evenly over the tortilla.

4.   Spread the bean mixture in the center of the tortilla. Fold the bottom and top ends of the tortilla in and roll up into a burrito.

5.   Microwave one more minute or until the burrito is heated through.

Per serving: 430 calories, 23.5 g protein, 53.5 g carbohydrate, 14.5 g fat, 7 grams saturated fat, 26 mg cholesterol, 8–10 g fiber, 480 mg sodium. Calories from fat: 30 percent.

Easy 3-Bean Salad
Makes four servings.

1 8.75-ounce can kidney beans, drained and rinsed (about 1 cup).
1 8.75-ounce can garbanzo beans, drained and rinsed (about 1 cup).
1 8.75-ounce can green or yellow wax beans, drained and rinsed (about 1 cup).
1/4 cup finely diced yellow or white onion.
4 Tbs. bottled vinaigrette (that uses olive oil or canola oil).
Add all the ingredients to a serving bowl. Toss well. This will store covered in the refrigerator for several days.
Per serving: 160 calories, 7 g protein, 27.5 g carbohydrate, 3 g fat, 0 g saturated fat, 0 mg cholesterol, 7 g fiber, 635 mg sodium. Calories from fat: 17 percent.

Sides, salads, sandwiches, and such

Spicy Hummus with Crudités and Crackers

This is a variation on the really tasty Middle Eastern dip/spread. You may have to search a bit to find tahini, although it is available in many supermarkets on the East and West Coasts.
Makes about three cups of dip.
1 15.5-oz. 50-percent-less sodium garbanzo beans.
3 cloves garlic, minced or pressed.
1/3 cup tahini (sesame seed paste).
1/4 cup lemon juice.
3 Tbs. light or fat-free sour cream.
2 Tbs. light cream cheese.
1/4 tsp. seasoning salt (optional).
1/4 tsp. ground cumin.
1/4 tsp. paprika.
2 Tbs. finely chopped fresh parsley (optional).
Crudités: choose crisp vegetables such as red bell pepper, carrots, celery, cauliflower, broccoli, green beans, and so on.
Crackers: choose from the many reduced-fat crackers on the market.
1. Drain the garbanzo beans and rinse well. (Reserve some of the liquid to add back if you need it to make a thinner dip.)
2. Place the beans, garlic, tahini, lemon juice, sour cream, cream cheese, seasoning salt, cumin, paprika, and parsley in a food

processor. Blend until somewhat smooth. Add more lemon juice or garbanzo liquid to taste. Use immediately or cover and refrigerate (it will keep for several days). Serve with vegetables and crackers.

Per serving: (1/3 cup dip) 100 calories, 1 g protein, 9 g carbohydrate, 5.5 g fat, 1 g saturated fat, 1 mg cholesterol, 3 g fiber, 120 mg sodium. Calories from fat: 50 percent.

When each serving is eaten with a cup of suggested vegetables, the fiber increases to about 6 grams per serving.

 # Lemon Dijon Salmon
Makes two servings.

2 salmon steaks (about 6 ounces each).
1 Tbs. Dijon mustard.
Garlic salt (about 1/2 tsp.).
Freshly ground pepper.
1/2 onion, thinly sliced.
1/2 lemon.
2 to 3 tsp. capers.

1. Preheat the oven to 400 degrees. Line a nine-inch pie plate with a large sheet of foil (enough so it can be wrapped back over the fish and sealed) and spray the foil generously with canola cooking spray. Lay salmon steaks in prepared pan.
2. Spread the fish steaks evenly with Dijon mustard.
3. Sprinkle the fish steaks with garlic salt and ground pepper to your liking.
4. Lay thinly sliced onion over the top.
5. Squeeze 1/2 lemon over the top of the salmon and sprinkle capers over the top.
6. Wrap the edges of the foil over the top of fish and seal the edges together. Bake about 15 minutes. Open the foil and let bake about five minutes more or until the salmon is cooked throughout.
7. Serve with steamed brown rice or cooked pasta and some vegetables.

Per serving: 231 calories, 30 g protein, 5 g carbohydrate, 10 g fat, 1.5 g saturated fat, 80 mg cholesterol, 1 g fiber, 678 mg sodium. Calories from fat: 39 percent.

Per serving (when each serving is served with 3/4 cup of steamed brown rice and a cup of broccoli): 475 calories, 38.5 g protein, 56 g carbohydrate, 11 g fat, 1.7

g saturated fat, 80 mg cholesterol, 8 g fiber, 720 mg sodium. Calories from fat: 21 percent. Omega-3 fatty acids: 1.5 g.

 # Simple Salmon Pasta Salad

This is one of my favorite salads. When I cook grilled salmon, I make extra on purpose so I can make this salad the next day with the leftovers.

Makes about two entrée servings.

Salmon:

2 cups whole wheat blend bow tie or rotelle pasta, cooked *al dente*.

1 cup salmon flakes (freshly cooked or grilled salmon fillets or steaks, broken into flakes with fork, with no bones or skin).

1 cup crisp-tender asparagus pieces, steamed or microwaved.

3 green onions, finely chopped.

Dressing:

1 Tbs. canola mayo or light mayonnaise.

2 Tbs. fat-free or light sour cream.

1 Tbs. lemon juice.

1 1/2 tsp. Dijon or prepared mustard.

1/2 tsp. dill weed.

Black pepper to taste.

1. Place the pasta, salmon, asparagus, and green onions in a serving bowl.
2. Blend the dressing ingredients until smooth. Add to pasta salad ingredients and stir to mix.

Per serving: 339 calories, 18 g protein, 45 g carbohydrate, 9.5 g fat, 1.5 g saturated fat, 29 mg cholesterol, 7 g fiber, 122 mg sodium. Calories from fat: 26 percent. Omega-3 fatty acid per serving: 1 g.

 # Easy Omega-3 Fatty Acid Tuna Sandwich

6 1/2 ounces albacore tuna, canned in spring water, drained.

1 Tbs. sweet or dill pickle relish (optional).

1/4 tsp. salt (optional).

1 Tbs. canola mayo or light mayonnaise.

1/2 Tbs. minced onion.

1/4 cup minced celery.

1 Tbs. light or fat-free sour cream.

Pepper to taste.

2 slices whole-wheat or whole-grain bread (toasted if desired).

Lettuce leaves and tomato slices.

1.   Combine the tuna, relish, salt, mayo, sour cream, onion, and celery in a small bowl; mix well. Add pepper to taste.

2.   Spread the mixture on slices of bread to make a sandwich. Add lettuce leaves, and tomato slices.

Per serving: 320 calories, 27 g protein, 34 g carbohydrate, 8.5 g fat, 1.4 g saturated fat, 27 mg cholesterol, 4.5 g fiber, 676 mg sodium. Calories from fat: 25 percent. There are about 0.5 g omega-3 fatty acids from tuna, and about 0.5 g from the canola mayonnaise.

Other quick entrées

Oat Bran Meat Loaf

This meatloaf tastes so much better than it sounds. Each serving contributes five grams of mostly soluble fiber to the meal too!

Makes five servings.

1 1/4 cup canned chick peas (garbanzo beans), drained and rinsed.

1/2 cup oat bran.

1/2 tsp. black pepper.

1/2 tsp. salt (optional).

2 cloves garlic, minced or pressed, or 1/2 teaspoon garlic powder.

1 Tbs. Worcestershire sauce.

2 Tbs. Heinz chili sauce.

1 Tbs. prepared mustard.

1 lb. ground sirloin (about 9-percent fat) or extra-lean ground beef.

1 cup grated, reduced-fat, sharp cheddar cheese (optional).

1 small onion, finely chopped.

Canola cooking spray.

1 cup tomato sauce.

1.   Preheat the oven to 350 degrees. Coat a 9-by-5-inch loaf pan with canola cooking spray.

2.   Add the ingredients up to and including mustard to a mixer or food processor. You can also mash with a pastry blender or potato masher.

3.   Process until well mixed (there will still be some lumps).

4.   If using a mixer, add beef, cheese, and onion to bean mixture and mix until well blended. If using a food processor, blend bean mixture

with beef, cheese, and onion with hands (or use a spoon) in a large mixing bowl.

5. Add the mixture to a pan and form into a loaf.
6. Bake for 30 minutes. Pour tomato sauce over the top and bake 15 minutes longer.

Per serving: 286 calories, 24.5 g protein, 28.5 g carbohydrate, 10 g fat, 3.5 g saturated fat, 33 mg cholesterol, 5 g fiber, 700 mg sodium. Calories from fat: 29 percent.

Light Club Sandwich

Makes one sandwich.

2 slices of Louis Rich turkey bacon.

2 slices of whole-wheat bread.

1 tsp. of canola mayonnaise or light mayo blended with 1 tsp. of light or fat-free sour cream.

2 lettuce leaves.

1 large slice turkey breast (about 2 ounces).

Pepper to taste.

1/2 large tomato, sliced.

1. Cook the bacon in a nonstick frying pan, over low heat, until crisp.
2. Spread one side of each bread slice lightly with mayonnaise mixture. Arrange lettuce leaf on one slice; top with one slice of turkey; sprinkle with pepper, then cover with another bread slice, mayonnaise side up. Top with another leaf of lettuce, tomato slices, bacon slices, and remaining bread slice, mayonnaise side down.
3. Cut the sandwich diagonally into fourths; secure each quarter with decorated toothpicks if desired.

Per serving: 350 calories, 19 g protein, 38 g carbohydrate, 12.5 g fat, 2.7 g saturated fat, 49 mg cholesterol, 5.5 g fiber, 1400 mg sodium. Calories from fat: 32 percent.

Homemade Napa Almond Chicken Salad Sandwich

To add a couple of servings of higher fiber and nutrient-rich whole grains, serve the chicken salad on two slices of 100-percent whole-grain bread or in a whole wheat pita pocket. You can even make a wrap sandwich using a whole-wheat flour tortilla.

Makes at least four sandwiches.
3 cups shredded roasted or rotisserie chicken, without skin.
1 cup red grapes cut in half.
2/3 cup finely chopped celery.
1/3 cup sliced almonds, honey roasted or plain roasted.
Dressing:
1/2 cup low fat or light mayonnaise (or nonfat Greek plain yogurt).
2 Tbs. honey.
2 Tbs. Dijon mustard.
1/4 tsp. black pepper.
Garnish (optional):
8 leaves of romaine lettuce.
8 slices of tomato.
Serve the chicken salad on whole wheat bread, tortilla, or pita.

1. In a medium-sized bowl, combine the shredded chicken, grapes, celery, and almonds.
2. In a small bowl, combine the dressing ingredients (light mayonnaise, honey, mustard, and pepper) with whisk or spoon until smooth and blended. Drizzle the dressing over the chicken and grape mixture and stir to blend.
3. Spoon the chicken mixture onto bread of choice to make at least four sandwiches, garnish with lettuce and tomato if desired and serve!

Per serving (if four per recipe): 500 calories, 42 g protein, 51 g carbohydrate, 14 g fat, 2.6 g saturated fat, 6 g monounsaturated fat, 5 g polyunsaturated fat, 96 mg cholesterol, 7 g fiber, 764 mg sodium. Calories from fat: 25 percent. Omega-3 fatty acids: 0.4 g. Omega-6 fatty acids: 4.5 g.

Berry and Blue Cheese Spinach Salad

This is truly one of my all time favorite salads—it just doesn't get old. Change it up and make it an entrée salad by adding grilled chicken or salmon.

Makes four servings.

8 cups fresh baby spinach leaves, packed (washed, rinsed, and dried well).
2 cups fresh berries (sliced strawberries, raspberries, or blackberries).
1/2 cup dried cranberries or dried blueberries (optional).
3/4 cup toasted walnut halves or pieces* (pecans or almonds can be substituted).
1/3 to 1/2 cup blue cheese, crumbled.
1/3 to 1/2 cup bottled light raspberry or pomegranate vinaigrette.

1. Place the spinach in a medium/large serving bowl. Top with berries, cranberries (if desired), toasted walnuts, and blue cheese.
2. Right before serving, drizzle the vinaigrette over the top and toss to blend well. Divide the mixture into four salad bowls or plates and serve!

* Toast the walnuts by placing them in a nonstick skillet (give a nice spray of canola or olive oil cooking spray if desired) and heat over medium heat, stirring often, until the walnuts are golden brown and fragrant.

Per serving: 280 calories, 10 g protein, 17 g carbohydrate, 17 g fat, 3.5 g saturated fat, 3 g monounsaturated fat, 10.5 g polyunsaturated fat, 8 mg cholesterol, 7 g fiber, 360 mg sodium. Omega-3 fatty acids: 2.2 g. Omega-6 fatty acids: 8.3 g.

 # Monounsaturated Side Salad

This salad is not just rich in monounsaturated fats—it's rich in fiber. **Makes four servings.**

1/2 avocado, cut into bite-size pieces.

1/2 cucumber, sliced.

1 cup chopped tomatoes or cherry tomatoes cut in half.

1 cup kidney beans (or 1/2 cup kidney beans and 1/2 cup garbanzo), drained and rinsed.

6 Tbs. Wish-Bone olive oil vinaigrette (or other dressing that uses olive oil or canola oil).

4 to 6 cups read-to-serve salad greens of your choice.

1. Place the avocado, cucumber, tomatoes, and beans into a serving bowl. Toss with dressing; set aside in the refrigerator until needed.
2. Right before mealtime, toss the vegetable mixture with lettuce.

Per serving: 155 calories, 6 g protein, 19 g carbohydrate, 7 g fat, 0.7 g saturated fat, 0 mg cholesterol, 7 g fiber, 460 mg sodium. Calories from fat: 43 percent.

Breakfast ideas

Light Denver Omelet for Two

I know this looks like it takes a bit of time, what with whipping the egg whites and everything, but once you know what you're doing, you can turn this out in 10 minutes. If you don't want to whip the egg whites, just beat them into the rest of the egg mixture (it won't be as fluffy, but it still tastes great).

Makes two servings.

Canola cooking spray.

1 cup sliced fresh mushrooms or other vegetable.

1 medium green pepper, chopped.

4 green onions, sliced diagonally.

1/4 tsp. dried basil.

1/2 cup chicken broth (water can also be used).

3 ounces (1/2 cup slightly heaping) lean ham, cut into 2-inch-long strips.

1/2 cup cherry tomatoes, halved (or other tomatoes).

1/2 cup egg substitute.

2 eggs, separated.

1. Coat a medium nonstick frying pan with canola cooking spray, and heat over medium heat. Add mushrooms, green pepper, green onions, and basil. Sauté for about 30 seconds, then pour in the chicken broth and cook, stirring frequently, until the vegetables are tender. Stir in ham and cherry tomatoes and cook for about a minute to heat through.
2. Blend the egg substitute and egg yolks in a medium-sized bowl and set aside. With mixer, beat the egg whites until stiff. Carefully fold the egg whites into egg-yolk mixture.
3. Coat a nonstick omelet pan or small nonstick frying pan with canola cooking spray (or use 1/2 tsp. canola oil or canola margarine), and heat over medium-low heat. Spread half of the egg mixture in a pan. Heat until the top looks firm (about two minutes). If your pan cooks hotter than normal (as some nonstick pans do), then cook over low heat. Flip the omelet over to lightly brown other side (about one minute).
4. Fill with half of the vegetable-ham filling, and fold as desired. Remove to serving plate. Repeat with the remaining egg mixture to make a second fluffy omelet.

Per serving: 190 calories, 9 g carbohydrate, 22 g protein, 7 g fat, 2 g saturated fat, 229 mg cholesterol, 2 g fiber, 690 mg sodium. Calories from fat: 35 percent.

 # Egg Muffin Sandwich Lite
Makes two sandwiches.

2 whole-grain English muffins, toasted.

1 egg.

1/4 cup egg substitute.

2 slices of Canadian bacon (or thick slices lean ham).

1 6.5-oz empty tuna can (or similar), washed, labels removed.

Freshly ground pepper.

2 slices of 1/3 low-fat American cheese (or similar).

Canola cooking spray.

1. Coat half of a nine-inch nonstick frying pan with canola cooking spray, and heat over medium heat.
2. In a small bowl, beat the egg with egg substitute; set aside.
3. Place Canadian bacon in the pan over the spray coated area. Spray the inside of the tuna can with canola cooking spray, and set the can on the other side of the pan to start heating. When the bottom side of the bacon is light brown, flip over to the other side and cook until light brown. Remove the slices from pan and set aside.
4. Pour half of the egg mixture (1/4 cup) into the tuna can. Sprinkle with freshly ground pepper to taste. When the surface of the egg begins to firm, cut around the inside of the can with a butter knife to free the edges. Turn the egg over with a cake fork, and cook one minute more.
5. Remove the egg from the can.
6. Coat the can with canola cooking spray. Repeat with the remaining egg.
7. To assemble, layer the English muffin bottom with a slice of cheese, then egg, a piece of Canadian bacon, and the English muffin top. To reheat, microwave each sandwich for 20 seconds on high.

Per serving: 287 calories, 21.5 g protein, 30.5 g carbohydrate, 9 g fat, 3.8 g saturated fat, 130 mg cholesterol, 5 g fiber, 1100 mg sodium. Calories from fat: 28 percent.

 # Sun-Dried Tomato Pesto Bagel Spread

Makes spread for about three bagels.

1/2 cup light or Neufchatel cream cheese.

1 clove garlic, minced or pressed.

1 Tbs. fresh basil leaves, fresh and chopped.

1 Tbs. julienne-style sun-dried tomatoes from bag, soaked in warm water until tender, then drained.

2 Tbs. pine nuts, pecans, or walnuts.

1. Add all ingredients to small food processor and process until well blended. Spread on bagels.

Per serving: (with whole grain bagel) 300 calories, 40 g carbohydrate, 14 g protein, 9 g fat, 4.5 g saturated fat, 20 mg cholesterol, 8 g fiber, 205 mg sodium. Calories from fat: 27 percent.

The Lox-ness Monster Bagel Spread

Makes about half a cup of spread (enough for about four bagels).
1/2 cup light cream cheese.
2 ounces lox, finely chopped.
1 green onion, finely chopped.
Pinch of fresh or dried dill (optional).
Pinch of capers (optional).

1. Blend all the ingredients in a food processor until well mixed. You should still be able to see some small pieces of lox. Spread on bagels.

Per serving (with whole-wheat bagel): 270 calories, 13 g protein, 38.5 g carbohydrate, 7 g fat, 3.5 g saturated fat, 18 mg cholesterol, 4 g fiber, 560 mg sodium. Calories from fat: 23 percent.

Apple Lover's Oatmeal

Makes one serving.
1 packet instant oatmeal, plain. (If you use flavored, sweetened instant oatmeal, such as "maple and brown sugar," then don't add the brown sugar.)
1 individual serving applesauce (3.9 oz), unsweetened (1/3 cup).
1 Tbs. brown sugar.
1/4 tsp. ground cinnamon.
1/2 cup low-fat milk (or similar—soy milk or almond milk can also be used).

1. In a large, microwave-safe soup bowl, blend all the ingredients together. Microwave on high for 1 1/2 minutes. Stir, then microwave for another 1 1/2 minutes. Serve hot.

Per serving: 180 calories, 5.5 g protein, 35 g carbohydrate, 2 grams fat, 0.8 g saturated fat, 5 mg cholesterol, 2.5 g fiber, 140 mg sodium. Calories from fat: 10 percent.

Note: To make a more balanced breakfast, enjoy this oatmeal with a strip or two of Louis Rich Turkey Bacon.

Oatmeal Raisin Bites

You can make a batch of these babies and then pop them in the freezer in a resealable plastic bag. Take out a cookie whenever you need one. They thaw quickly in the microwave or at room temperature.

Makes 32 large cookies.

6 Tbs. canola margarine or butter, softened.
6 Tbs. fat-free or light cream cheese.
1 cup packed brown sugar.
1/2 cup granulated sugar.
1/4 cup low-fat buttermilk.
1/4 cup egg substitute.
2 Tbs. maple syrup.
2 Tbs. vanilla extract.
1 cup of whole-wheat flour (unbleached flour can be used).
1/2 tsp. baking soda.
1 1/2 tsp. ground cinnamon.
1/4 tsp. salt.
2 cups quick or old-fashioned oats.
1 cup raisins.
1/2 cup chopped walnuts (optional).

1. Preheat the oven to 350 degrees. Coat two cookie sheets with canola cooking spray. In a large bowl, beat the butter with cream cheese. Beat in the sugars, buttermilk, egg substitute, maple syrup, and vanilla until light and fluffy.
2. Combine the flour, baking soda, cinnamon, and salt; beat into the butter mixture.
3. Stir in the oats, raisins, and nuts if desired, mixing well.
4. Use a cookie scoop (or drop by rounded tablespoonfuls) to form cookies and place two inches apart on the prepared cookie sheets. For flatter (rather than rounded) cookies, press each cookie mound down lightly with a spoon, spatula, or your fingers.
5. Bake one cookie sheet at a time, in the upper third of the oven for about 10 minutes, or until lightly browned. Remove the cookies to the wire racks to cool completely. Store in an airtight container.

Per serving: 120 calories, 2 g protein, 22 g carbohydrate, 3 g fat, 0.4 g saturated fat, 5 mg cholesterol, 2 g fiber, 36 mg sodium. Calories from fat: 22 percent.

Chapter 6

Navigating the Supermarket

It's easy to get confused while shopping in the trenches (a.k.a. your typical grocery store). Each product label that catches your eye inevitably hits you with countless advertising slogans and nutrition terms. Just remember, the bottom line is that all these companies are basically trying to sell you something; they all want a piece of your food budget. The package might boast "sugar-free" or "fat-free," but it's the nutrition information label that's going to tell you whether that product has just as many grams of carbohydrates or just as many calories as the regular products.

It's also the nutrition information label that is going to indicate what the company considers the serving size to be. The serving size of many individual or small frozen pizzas is one-third of the "small" pizza. There are some reduced-fat ice cream bars out there that, when you check the label, still contain more than 13 grams of fat per serving. The moral of this story is to read your labels. You'll get the information you need for counting and calculating from the nutrition information label—check the portion size, the grams of fat, carbohydrates, and calories when shopping for and comparing food products.

The second lesson is a bit more difficult to master. Some of us may be using these fat-free products as an excuse to overeat. I don't think we are entirely to blame here. If these products aren't as satisfying, we're probably more likely to keep on eating and eating in the hope of reaching some level of satisfaction. Also, some of the advertising has basically encouraged us to eat as much as we want—after all, it's fat-free! So select light and fat-free products that you truly like—that taste satisfying to you—and that you can eat in modest serving sizes. Otherwise, they aren't going to do any good for your health and enjoyment.

Avoiding the land mines

Have you ever noticed that the nutrition facts information on the label of a baking mix or cake mix is listed in two columns? It usually gives two sets of information, one for *Mix* and one for *Baked* (or, *As Prepared*). Normally, they will give you two amounts of fat grams; one from the mix and one for the total amount of fat per serving after it's prepared. This is important information, because many of these mixes call for a one-third cup of oil, three eggs, or a stick of butter.

Several companies have started giving only the grams of fat in the mix. If you look real closely, which is what I get paid to do, you'll see a tiny asterisk next to the grams of fat. Then you look down at the very bottom of the label and, in small print, it reads something like this: "Amount in mix."

They do give you the daily percentage value for grams of fat "as prepared," but let's face it, what does that really mean to most people? Most people just quickly scan the label until they see grams of fat. I can just hear people thinking, *Oh, goody, four grams of fat!* When, in reality, if they follow the directions on the box, a serving has something more like nine or 13 grams of fat per serving.

Just so you know what to watch out for, here is an example:

A serving of Pillsbury Thick 'n Fudgy Cheesecake Swirl Deluxe Brownie Mix contains 4.5 grams of fat. When you follow the directions on the box, adding a one-fourth cup of oil and two eggs to the mix, the grams of fat per serving increases to nine grams of fat. But you won't see nine grams anywhere on the label. If you look really hard, you'll find 14 percent daily value for fat in the "prepared" column. You have to do a little math to get to nine from the 14 percent daily value given on the label.

It's all in a name

We've come to rely on certain brands with diet-sounding names to steer us toward the better choices where our waistlines and diabetes are concerned. Weight Watchers, Lean Cuisine, and Slim Fast, for example, are all music to the ears. But don't let those seductive names fool you. Some of these products are just as high in calories, fat, and carbohydrate grams as the overtly "sinful" products farther down the aisle.

In many cases, what they are selling you is portion control and a pretty name (for a handsome price). Keep your eyes open and read the label!

Fat-free, but full of calories

Here's a news flash—just because a product is fat-free doesn't mean it is calorie-free or that you can eat the whole box in one sitting. In fact, many of these fat-free products have just as many calories as the full-fat versions. How can that be? In a word—*sugar*. Sugar, whether it comes from honey, corn syrup, brown sugar, or high-fructose corn syrup, can add moisture and help tenderize bakery products. When added to foods such as ice cream, it adds flavor and structure. So I'm not surprised that manufacturers have turned to sugar for assistance while developing reduced-fat and fat-free products.

The majority of the fat-free and lower-fat products on the supermarket shelves only offer us average savings of 10 or 20 calories per serving. Does this mean we shouldn't buy any of these products? Sort of. It's best to eat mostly whole unprocessed foods. But for the times we do buy these packaged products we need to still enjoy eating them, watch our serving size, and keep track of the grams of carbohydrates we are taking in.

Taking a tour of your supermarket

Next time you walk around your supermarket, aisle by aisle, look for smarter foods and products that offer:

- Lower-carbohydrate, lower-sugar, and reduced-calorie products that might come in handy when you are trying to balance a meal or snack.
- Good, easy sources of soluble fiber (and fiber in general).
- Products and foods that feature the smart fats—omega-3 fatty acids and monounsaturated fats.
- Whole-grain products that contribute fiber and other nutrients, and which have a positive effect on your blood sugar.

I've included some product information for some of the food/product categories that I thought might help you the most.

Choosing a healthy breakfast cereal

The cereal aisle is a long one, full of contradictions. You'll find cereals made with refined grains with nearly no fiber, and cereals made with whole grains and bran, boasting seven grams or more of fiber. There are cereals with so much sugar they seem more like boxes of little cookies. And, luckily, there are cereals with sugar listed far down on the ingredient list.

Choosing a healthy breakfast cereal is mainly about getting more whole grains and less sugar. There's no excuse not to get at least one serving of whole grains if you eat cereal for breakfast. And it's well worth the effort; recent research suggests those who eat more whole grains and foods rich in cereal fiber are at lower risk of obesity, type 2 diabetes, and heart disease.

Cereals made with refined grains have generally not been linked to health benefits, such as a lower risk of death from heart disease, as whole-grain breakfast cereals have. Refined-grain cereals do not lower the risk of gaining weight or having a higher BMI (body mass index), but whole grain-rich cereals do.

Taste or nutrition?

Of course, one person's perfect whole-grain cereal with less sugar is another person's bowl of sawdust. If you like breakfast cereals that come in lots of colors and artificial flavors, then, yes, you probably do have to choose between taste and nutrition. But if you like a cereal with natural flavors from toasted whole grains, and maybe some nuts and dried fruit, you'll have many healthful cereals to choose from.

And, yes, dried fruits do add nutrition to your cereal. A quarter of a cup of raisins, for example, has about one and a half grams of fiber plus four percent of the Recommended Daily Value for vitamin E and about six percent each of the Daily Value for vitamins B-1, B-6, and iron, magnesium, and selenium. But when you look on the nutrition facts label for Raisin Bran, for example, you might be shocked to see there are 19 grams of sugar in a one-cup serving. What's going on is that any sugars—even those from natural sources such as dried fruit—are counted in the sugar grams listed on the label.

Focus on the grams of carbohydrates per serving of the cereal, because this is going to be what you count in your carbohydrate budget for that meal.

Does bran matter?

Bran's biggest benefit is boosting the number of grams of fiber per serving. This makes the cereal seem more filling, both in the short run in a couple hours. This staying power may have something to do with the lower glycemic index of bran cereals. One study noted that the glycemic index of corn flakes was more than twice that of bran cereal.

Other recent research found that adding bran to the diet reduced the risk of weight gain in men aged 40–75. Another study, in women aged 38–63, reported that as intake of fiber and whole-grain foods went up, the rate of weight gain tended to decrease. Eating refined grains had the opposite effect: as the intake of refined-grain foods increased, so did weight gain.

How much sugar?

Does the ingredients list for your cereal look a lot like that on, say, a box of cookies? One ounce of Mini Oreo cookies has 11 grams of sugar and 130 calories

(34 percent of its calories come from sugar). And sugar is the second ingredient listed (enriched flour is first). Many cereals have ingredient lists that look similar—such as Cookie Crisp Cereal, with 44 percent of calories from sugar.

The U.S. Government's Dietary Reference Intakes recommend that added sugars not exceed 25 percent of total calories (to ensure sufficient intake of micronutrients). And though there isn't a specific guideline for cereal, it makes sense to aim for a cereal that gets 25 percent or less of its calories from sugar. (If the cereal contains dried fruit, this could be a tad higher.)

To calculate the percentage of calories from sugar in your cereal:
1. Multiply the grams of sugar per serving by four (there are four calories per gram of sugar).
2. Divide this number (calories from sugar) by the total number of calories per serving.
3. Multiply this number by 100 to get the percentage of calories from sugar.

Though you can find plenty of cereals with five grams of fiber per serving or more, some of them go a little bit over the "25 percent of calories from sugar" guideline. But if the percentage of sugar calories is still below 30 percent, the first ingredient is a whole grain, and the cereal tastes good, it may still be a good choice overall.

Kashi GoLean Crunch Honey Almond Flax has eight grams of fiber and 12 grams of sugar per serving (24 percent of calories from sugar). The first three ingredients are Kashi Seven Whole Grains and Sesame blend (whole oats, long-grain brown rice, rye, hard red winter wheat, triticale, buckwheat, barley, sesame seeds); soy flakes, and brown rice syrup. This is basically a kashi-fied version of granola, and three grams of the eight grams of fiber is from soluble fiber (thanks to the oats and barley).

Eight good-tasting picks

After some taste testing and input from cereal lovers, I came up with eight picks for the best-tasting healthful breakfast cereals. The cereals on my list had to have a whole grain as the first ingredient and at least five grams of fiber per serving. Sugar had to be around 25 percent of calories from sugar or less, unless dried fruit was among the top three ingredients. I also tried to choose cereals that would probably go over with most of you and that are easily found in most supermarkets.

- **Post Grape-Nuts Cranberry Vanilla Fit:** 2/3 cup equals 220 calories, 44 g carbs, 5 g fiber, 9 g sugar, 6 g protein and 16 percent of calories from sugar. The first three ingredients are whole-grain wheat flour, whole grain puffed barley, and dried cranberries, whole-grain oats, and brown sugar.

- **Fiber One Honey Clusters**: 1 cup equals 170 calories, 44 g carbs, 10 g fiber, 9 g sugar, 4 g protein, and 21 percent of calories from sugar. The first three ingredients are whole-grain wheat, corn bran, and wheat bran.

- **Quaker Oatmeal Squares**: 1 cup equals 210 calories, 44 g carbs, 5 g fiber, 9 g sugar, 6 g protein, and 17 percent of calories from sugar. The first three ingredients are whole-oat flour, whole-wheat flour, and brown sugar.

- **Shredded wheat:** 1 cup equals 170 calories, 40 g carbs, 6 g fiber, 0 g sugar, 6 g protein, and 0 percent of calories from sugar. The only ingredient is 100 percent whole grain cereal. I enjoy this with added fresh or dried fruit and nuts. If you opt for the frosted variety, it has 6 grams fiber and gets 23 percent of its calories from sugar.

- **Frosted Mini-Wheats**: 1 cup equals 200 calories, 47 g carbs, 6 g fiber, 11 g sugar, 5 g protein, and 22 percent of calories from sugar. The first three ingredients are whole-grain wheat, sugar, and high-fructose corn syrup.

- **Kellogg's Raisin Bran:** 1 cup equals 190 calories, 46 g carbs, 7 g fiber, 18 g sugar, 5 g protein, and 37 percent of calories from sugar. The first three ingredients are whole wheat, raisins, and wheat bran. Sugar is listed fourth in the ingredient list, but many of the calories from sugar come from the raisins.

- **Kashi Heart to Heart Honey Toasted Oat Cereal:** 3/4 cup equals 120 calories, 26 g carbs, 5 g fiber, 5 g sugar, 3 g protein, and 17 percent of calories from sugar. The first three ingredients are whole-oat flour, evaporated cane juice syrup, and oat bran. This is a higher-fiber alternative to Cheerios. I think they taste better too.

- **Wheat Chex:** 3/4 cup equals 160 calories, 39 g carbs, 6 g fiber, 5 g sugar, 5 g protein, and 12.5 percent of calories from sugar. The first three ingredients are whole-grain wheat, sugar, and salt.

- **Post Great Grains Protein Blend:** 1 cup equals 230 calories, 39 g carbs, 7 g fiber, 9 g sugar, 8 g protein, and 16 percent of calories from sugar. The first three ingredients are whole-grain wheat, whole-grain barley, and whole grain oats.

Diabetic-friendly frozen entrées

Frozen entrées come in handy in many situations—as a quick lunch during the workweek and as an easy dinner if you live alone or with one other person.

The problem with frozen entrées is that the ones that are lower in fat are almost always too low in calories and carbohydrates, and meager in the vegetable department. Many contain around 300 calories, the amount of calories in one measly bagel. In order to make the entrées satisfying, I found myself adding vegetables and/or nuts, cooked rice or noodles, or grated cheese. And if people are eating them as their complete meal, they are also totally devoid of fruit. Some frozen entrées are brimming with sodium. The companies taste-test products with the average American's taste preferences in mind, and guess what? The average American likes salt.

You can add an extra half cup of whole grain noodles or brown rice, half-cup of steamed vegetables, and a piece or two of fruit to help round out the entrées, which is what I did when I was trying each of the entrées listed on the following page. But this is sort of defeating the purpose of a frozen entrée, isn't it? I listed the nutrition information of some of the frozen entrées I found interesting in my supermarket.

Because some people with type 2 diabetes fare better with a little more fat in their meal (preferably monounsaturated fat), I included any non-"light" entrée that seemed workable.

Brand/Meal	Calories	Carbs (g)	Fat (g)	Protein (g)	Fiber (g)	Sodium (mg)
Healthy Choice						
Golden roasted turkey breast	270	38	4	19	7	520
Chicken parmigiana	340	49	9	16	7	580
Country herb chicken	250	34	5	16	6	500
Lemon pepper fish	330	58	4	14	4	530
Chicken enchilada suprema	300	46	7	13	4	560

Brand/Meal	Calories	Carbs (g)	Fat (g)	Protein (g)	Fiber (g)	Sodium (mg)
Lean Cuisine						
Steak tips portabello	150	14	4	15	2	570
Chicken carbonara	240	29	6	18	2	660
Chicken with basil cream sauce	230	28	5	19	2	490
Salmon with basil	250	38	2.5	19	4	500
Roasted tur-key breast	290	38	7	19	3	890
Ranchero braised beef	250	32	6	16	2	610
Amy's						
Mexican cas-serole bowl	380	48	16	12	8	780
Kashi						
Spicy black bean enchilada	260	45	7	8	8	600
Lemongrass coconut chicken	300	38	8	18	7	680
Marie Callender's						
Beef pot roast	320	35	11	20	6	760
Steak and roasted potatoes	350	40	11	22	6	930

Saturated fat for all items is between 1 and 9 mg.

Dairy products

We need milk to keep our cereal company, to help liquefy our pancake batter, and to lighten our coffee. The great thing about milk is you can take out some of the fat and saturated fat and still have milk that does all the things you want it to do. And as you remove the fat, the cholesterol goes too.

- Milk goes from 35 mg cholesterol in a cup of whole milk down to 15 mg in a cup of one-percent milk.

- Cottage cheese goes from 25 mg cholesterol in a half cup of small curd cottage cheese down to 10 mg in low-fat.

- It gets a little tricky with other dairy products. When you take the fat out of cheese, for example, if you start going past the halfway mark, it starts looking and tasting a lot less like cheese and a lot more like plastic.

No matter the amount of fat, most dairy products should be consumed in sensible amounts; they all need to be counted into your daily totals, because many such as milk and yogurt contribute carbohydrate grams galore. Then, the other dairy products that are low in carbohydrates need to be counted, because they are most likely contributing some fat and/or protein grams (such as cheese). Either way, you want to make sure you are counting them to see how they help balance your meals or snacks and what effect they have on your blood sugar in certain amounts.

Food Item	Calories	Carbs (g)	Fat (g)	Protein (g)	Fiber (g)	Sodium (mg)
Milk (1 cup)						
Skim milk	90	13	0	9	0	130
Low-fat milk (1%)	120	14	2.5	11	1.5	160
Low-fat milk (2%)	130	13	5	10	3	140
Whole milk	150	13	8	8	5	125
Cottage cheese (1/2 cup)						

Food Item	Calories	Carbs (g)	Fat (g)	Protein (g)	Fiber (g)	Sodium (mg)
Low-fat cottage cheese (2%)	90	4	2.5	13	0	410
Fat-free cottage cheese	80	5	0	14	0	420
Yogurt						
Nonfat Greek, plain (8 ounces)	130	13	0	19	0	130
Vanilla Greek (8 ounces)	180	23	0	21	0	100
"Light" fat-free, flavored yogurts (6 ounces)	90	15	0	5	0	75
99% fat-free flavored yogurts (6 ounces)	170	33	2	5	1	80
Low-fat custard-style, flavored yogurt (6 ounces)		190	32	3	8	2
Sour Cream (2 Tbs.)						
Fat-free sour cream	20	3	0	1	0	40
Light sour cream	40	2	2.5	2	0	25

High monounsaturated fat salad dressings and spreads

The products listed here mainly contain the high monounsaturated fat vegetable oils: canola oil, olive oil, or a combination of the two.

Food Item	Calories	Carbs (g)	Fat (g)
Mayonnaise: 1 Tbs.*			
Smart Balance Omega Light Mayo Dressing	50	2	5
Kraft Reduced Fat Mayonnaise with Olive Oil	35	2	3
Best Foods Canola	40	1	4
Best Foods with Olive Oil	60	1	6
Salad dressing: 2 Tbs.**			
Brianna's Blush Wine Vinaigrette	120	14	7
Dijon Honey Mustard	150	8	14
Ken's Steak House			
Lite Caesar	70	3	6
Lite Raspberry Walnut Vinaigrette	80	7	6
Hidden Valley Farmhouse Originals			

Food Item	Calories	Carbs (g)	Fat (g)
Pomegranate Vinaigrette	60	3	6
Italian with Herbs	80	3	7
Wish Bone			
Balsamic Vinaigrette	60	3	5
Newman's Own			
Olive Oil and Vinegar	150	1	16

*Mayonnaise: 80 or less mg sodium and 1 g saturated fat per serving.

**Salad dressing: Between 230 and 480 mg sodium and 1 g saturated fat per serving.

Chapter 7

Restaurant Rules to Eat By

Most health-conscious people go to restaurants and try to steer clear of one thing—overtly high-fat, high-calorie menu selections. But people with diabetes often have a few more things they worry about when approaching the menu. You need to get a feel for how many carbohydrate grams you might be eating and whether your selection is something that tends to keep your after-meal blood sugar high or not. You want to choose something that contributes a moderate amount of monounsaturated fat, because many find that this helps with blood sugar control. You will also be trying to keep saturated fat and trans fatty acids low and omega-3 fatty acids high, to help protect your heart. Many of you also need to count protein and potassium if you are on dialysis.

That's quite a bit to have on your plate (so to speak). All this could very well take the fun out of eating out. The trick is finding the happy medium between counting what you need to count and ordering and enjoying foods you like. It can be done; it takes a little practice. And the fact that many restaurant chains now list the grams of fat, fiber, and carbohydrates on their menu certainly helps too. Some of the suggested foods in this chapter have higher amounts of sodium than others, so if your doctor or dietitian has told you to limit sodium, make sure to consider that.

Cutting saturated fat and calories when eating out

Remember, some people with diabetes control their blood sugar better if they aren't on a very low-fat diet, but are on a moderate-fat diet (around 30 to 35 percent of calories from fat). If you are in this group, it is particularly important that you choose monounsaturated fats and omega-3 and omega-9 fatty acids whenever possible. No matter which group you are in, though, you will want to avoid foods high in animal fats, which load on extra calories and saturated fat. One of the downfalls of eating out is the hefty portions of meat and dairy they often serve you. There are a few things you can do to keep this in check:

- The lean cuts of beef at restaurants include filet mignon, sirloin, sirloin tips, or chopped sirloin, whereas the fattier cuts are ribeye, prime rib, porterhouse, and T-bone.

- Trim any visible fat from any cut of meat you order.

- Make sure your meat dish is accompanied by lots of vegetables (beans when possible). The vegetables will help fill you up so you won't be tempted to overdo the meat, and the vegetables and beans help boost fiber totals too (good for your health and your blood sugar).

- Order the kid-size burger or quarter-pounder instead of the third- or half-pound hamburger, and load up on lettuce, tomato, ketchup, and mustard, instead of mayonnaise, special sauces, and cheese.

- Order the petite or junior portions of meat, prime rib, and steaks when available.

- Automatically cut your steak, pork chop, ham, or roasted chicken in half and take the rest home for tomorrow's sandwich.

- Ask the restaurant to make your three-egg omelet with egg substitute, or one egg blended with three egg whites.

- Avoid extra cheese and try to keep your servings of heavy cheese dishes (pizza, cheese enchiladas, lasagna, and so on) moderate.

To avoid excessive calories in general, you basically need to avoid ordering foods made with *a lot* of:

- **Butter or margarine:** Each tablespoon of butter contains 11.5 grams of fat and 102 calories.

- **Mayonnaise:** Each tablespoon of mayonnaise contains 11 grams of fat and 100 calories. Creamy mayonnaise-based salad dressings are dripping with fat grams. Remember, one restaurant ladle adds up to two tablespoons of dressing, worth around 25 grams of fat.

- **Cream:** One-quarter cup of liquid whipping cream contains 22 grams of fat and 205 calories.

- **Oil:** Each tablespoon of oil contains 14 grams of fat and 120 calories. Avoid deep-fried anything, even if it is something healthful such as chicken or seafood. Have it grilled instead.

- **Sugar:** It is loaded with calories. It's not that you can't have any, but it helps to split the dessert you want to try with someone at the table or eat half and bring the other half home.

Healthier fast food? Really?

If you only have a few minutes or a few bucks, fast food can come in handy. It's true that fruits, vegetables, and fiber tend to be scarce in fast-food meals, but diabetes-friendly choices can be had at every fast-food chain; it's all in what and how you order!

Keep these six suggestions in mind

#1: Count the carbs. There's plenty of information about counting carbs in Chapter 4, so I know that you know all about it. This is just a reminder to count the carbs when you are eating in restaurants and fast-food chains so you can stick to your carbohydrate budget as much as practically possible for that meal.

#2: Start with healthful fast-food entrées like grilled chicken sandwiches or wraps, grilled chicken salads, and entrées based on beans or lean turkey or beef. It makes sense that the bigger the burger, the bigger the calorie and fat totals, so if you are a "double double" type of guy or gal, try to make it a single and fill in the space with produce like lettuce, tomato, and onion.

#3: Be cautious about condiments and extras. Half of the fat grams in many fast-food sandwiches come from the creamy sauces, spreads, or mayo added. Some condiments add a lot of fat and calories, though others are lower in calories and add no fat grams (but they will add some sodium) such as ketchup, marinara, mustard, and BBQ sauce.

Half of a packet of BBQ sauce or honey mustard sauce from most fast-food chains, for example, will add about 23 calories and no fat grams. Compare that to a tablespoon of mayonnaise with 90 calories and 10 grams of fat. Extras like cheese and bacon will rack on the calories and fat as well. Some burgers come with two slices of cheese in addition to bacon and/or onion rings.

#4: Watch out for the side dishes. Look for something colorful and fresh to keep your entrée company instead of something crispy and deep fried. Fresh fruit cups, yogurt parfaits, or side salads (using half a packet of the vinaigrette-type dressings) will do the trick. If you must have the french fries or onion rings and try to stick with the smallest size (and you can even share it with someone).

#5: Beverage calories count too. Pair your healthful entrée with water (which is what your body wants and needs) or with a beverage that either contributes key nutrients, like low-fat milk, or contributes flavor with zero or low calories, like unsweetened iced tea. If you're a soda lover, consider a low- or no-calorie option like Diet Coke with your meal. Or, if you prefer the taste of regular soda, consider a smaller sized portion.

Super soda tip: In some fast food restaurants, they hand you a cup to serve yourself with a beverage. In this case, you can add a splash of regular Coke or Dr. Pepper to your Diet Coke for a little added flavor punch with only a few added calories.

#6: Eat mindfully and in moderation. No matter which items you choose, any food or beverage can be part of a healthy diet when consumed mindfully and in moderation. Eating mindfully—no matter where we're eating—involves paying attention to hunger and satisfaction, being aware of and curious about why we are eating when we aren't hungry, and learning from it. And mostly, eating mindfully means breathing deeply and being in gratitude before starting our meal, eating slowly, and allowing ourselves to taste, savor, and find joy in every bite or sip.

With these six suggestions in mind, here are some examples of healthier fast-food options!

Slimmer sandwiches

- **KFC Honey BBQ Sandwich:** 320 calories, 3.5 g fat, 1 g saturated fat, 70 mg cholesterol, 770 mg sodium, 3 g fiber, 47 grams carbohydrate, 24 g protein.

- **Chick-fil-A Char grilled Chicken Sandwich:** 290 calories, 4 g fat, 1 g saturated fat, 60 mg cholesterol, 780 mg sodium, 3 g fiber, 36 g of carbohydrate, 28 g of protein.

- **Carl's Jr. Charbroiled BBQ Chicken Sandwich:** 390 calories, 7 g fat, 1.5 g saturated fat, 60 mg cholesterol, 990 mg sodium, 3 g fiber, 50 g of carbohydrate, 30 g of protein.

- **Wendy's Ultimate Grill Sandwich:** 370 calories, 7 g fat, 1.5 g saturated fat, 95 mg cholesterol, 880 mg sodium, 3 g fiber, 43 g carbohydrate, 34 g protein.

- **McDonald's Grilled Chicken Classic Sandwich:** 350 calories, 9 g fat, 2 g saturated fat, 65 mg cholesterol, 820 mg sodium, 3 g fiber, 42 g carbohydrate, 28 g protein.

- **Burger King Veggie Burger without mayo:** 320 calories, 7 g fat, 1 g saturated fat, 0 mg cholesterol, 960 mg sodium, 7 g fiber, 43 g carbohydrate, 22 g protein.

- **Burger King Tender Grill Chicken Sandwich without mayo:** 400 calories, 11 g fat, 2 g saturated fat, 70 mg cholesterol, 1260 mg sodium, 2 g fiber, 43 g carbohydrate, 31 g protein.

Better burgers

- **In-n-Out Hamburger (with onion and mustard and ketchup instead of spread):** 310 calories, 10 g fat, 4 g saturated fat, 35 mg cholesterol, 730 mg sodium, 3 g fiber, 41 g carbohydrate, 16 g protein.

- **Wendy's Jr. Hamburger:** 250 calories, 10 g fat, 4 g saturated fat, 40 mg cholesterol, 600 mg sodium, 2 g fiber, 25 g carbohydrate, 14 g protein.

- **Carl's Jr. Teriyaki Turkey Burger:** 470 calories, 14 g fat, 5 g saturated fat, 80 mg cholesterol, 1120 mg sodium, 3 g fiber, 55 g carbohydrate, 32 g protein.

- **McDonald's Grilled Onion Cheddar Burger:** 310 calories, 13 g fat, 6 g saturated fat, 40 mg cholesterol, 660 mg sodium, 2 g fiber, 33 g carbohydrate, 15 g protein.

- **Whopper Jr. (without mayo):** 260 calories, 10 g fat, 4 g saturated fat, 25 mg cholesterol, 440 mg sodium, 2 g fiber, 28 g carbohydrate, 13 g protein.

Wraps and such

- **Taco Bell Fresco Style Bean Burrito:** 350 calories, 9 g fat, 2.5 g saturated fat, 0 mg cholesterol, 950 mg sodium, 9 g fiber, 54 g carbohydrate, 12 g protein.

- **Wendy's Grilled Chicken Go Wrap:** 260 calories, 10 g fat, 3.5 g saturated fat, 55 mg cholesterol, 740 mg sodium, 1 g fiber, 25 g carbohydrate, 19 g protein.

- **McDonalds Chipotle BBQ Snack Wrap (grilled):** 250 calories, 8 g fat, 3.5 g saturated fat, 40 mg cholesterol, 670 mg sodium, 1 g fiber, 27 g carbohydrate, 16 grams protein.

- **Taco Bell Fresco Style Steak Burrito Supreme:** 350 calories, 9 g fat, 3 g saturated fat, 20 mg cholesterol, 990 mg sodium, 7 g fiber, 51 g carbohydrate, 17 g protein.

- **Jack in the Box Chicken Fajita Pita (made with whole grain but no salsa):** 320 calories, 11 g fat, 5 g saturated fat, 65 mg cholesterol, 870 mg sodium, 4 g fiber, 33 g carbohydrate, 24 g protein.

- **Chick-fil-A Char Grilled Chicken Cool Wrap:** 410 calories, 10 g fat, 4 g saturated fat, 60 mg cholesterol, 1070 mg sodium, 7 g fiber, 50 g carbohydrate, 32 g protein.

- **Wendy's Large Chili:** 270 calories, 8 g fat, 3 g saturated fat, 40 mg cholesterol, 1180 mg sodium, 7 g fiber, 31 g carbohydrate, 19 g protein.

Tasty entrée salads

- **Chick-fil-A Char Grilled Chicken and Fruit Salad (with reduced fat berry balsamic vinaigrette):** 330 calories, 9.5 g fat, 3.5 g saturated fat, 60 mg cholesterol, 700 mg sodium, 5 g fiber, 41 g carbohydrate, 22 g protein.
- **McDonalds Southwest Salad with Grilled Chicken (includes cilantro lime glaze and a southwest vegetable/bean blend):** 290 calories, 8 g fat, 2.5 g saturated fat, 70 mg cholesterol, 650 mg sodium, 7 g fiber, 28 g carbohydrate, 27 g protein.
- **Carl's Jr. Charbroiled Chicken Salad (with low-fat balsamic dressing):** 290 calories, 13 g fat, 4.5 g saturated fat, 40 mg cholesterol, 870 mg sodium, 3 g fiber, 28 g carbohydrate, 18 g protein.
- **Wendy's Apple Pecan Chicken Salad Half-Size (with roasted pecans and pomegranate dressing):** 340 calories, 18 g fat, 4.5 g saturated fat, 55 mg cholesterol, 710 mg sodium, 4 g fiber, 28 g carbohydrate, 19 g protein.

Elaine's top picks at a few restaurant chains

What about restaurants? When I was growing up, we went to a restaurant when it was somebody's birthday. People today go to restaurants weekly if not daily. The good news is no matter where you go, there are usually healthier menu options for people with type 2 diabetes—items with the lowest amount of saturated fat, calories, and sodium while offering higher amounts of protein and fiber.

Granted, options are changing all the time, particularly at fast food chains, but at the time I'm writing this Anniversary Edition, the following are a handful of my go-to options at some of America's restaurant chains.

TGI Fridays

Even if you don't have one of these restaurants in your town, it's a good example of what the better options might be at a standard American restaurant.

Salad

Friday's House Salad with bread stick and low fat balsamic vinaigrette: 290 calories, 3 g saturated fat, 10 g total fat, 570 mg sodium. Nutrition: 45 g carbs, 8 g protein, 4 g fiber.

Appetizer (individual)

BBQ Chicken Flatbread: 460 calories, 8 g saturated fat, 21 g total fat, 980 mg sodium. Nutrition: 44 g carbs, 23 g protein, 3 g fiber.

Appetizer (taste and share menu)

Thai Pork Tacos: 280 calories, 3.5 g saturated fat, 14 g total fat, 690 mg sodium. Nutrition: 25 g carbs, 14 g protein, 2 g fiber.

Entrées

Dragonfire Salmon: 600 calories, 9 g saturated fat, 34 grams total fat, 1980 mg sodium. Nutrition: 46 g carbs, 42 g protein, 6 g fiber.

Korean Steak Tacos (half order): 520 calories, 1.8 g saturated fat, 14.5 g total fat, 790 mg sodium. Nutrition: 79 g carbs, 19.5 g protein, 3.5 g fiber.

Bruschetta Chicken Pasta (half of the order): 460 calories, 4 g saturated fat, 21 g total fat, 1030 mg sodium. Nutrition: 45 g carbs, 23.5 g protein, 3 g fiber.

Hibachi Chicken Skewers (half order): 665 calories, 2.5 g saturated fat, 20.5 g total fat, 2380 mg sodium (lower the sodium by not using any of the dipping sauce served with it). Nutrition: 93 g carbs, 28 g protein, 4 grams fiber.

Jack Daniel's Grill Chicken and Shrimp: 570 calories, 2.5 g saturated fat, 11 g total fat, 2630 mg sodium. Nutrition: 77 g carbs, 44 g protein, 3 g fiber.

Kid's Menu

Grownups can order from the Kid's Menu too!

Chicken Skewer with grilled pita: 320 calories, 2 g saturated fat, 10 g total fat, 1000 mg sodium. Nutrition: 33 g carbs, 23 g protein, 2 g fiber.

Chicken Sandwich: 280 calories, 3.5 g saturated fat, 13 g total fat, 550 mg sodium. Nutrition: 24 g carbs, 14 g protein, 1 g fiber.

The steakhouse chain

There are many steakhouse chains across the country, and most of them do *not* provide any nutrition information for their interested patrons. Hopefully, it's obvious to avoid the gigantic, battered, deep-fried onion, which, rumor has it, contains more than 100 grams of fat.

Even if you avoid everything that is deep-fried (not just because of the fat and calories, but because anything deep-fried seems to cause high blood sugar for many people), what about the other items? If you want to have steak, which selections are best for you? There are a few things, no matter which steakhouse you're in, that will help put you in the nutritional driver's seat:

- Ask the chef to cook your meat without butter or added fat.
- Order your meat in small portions or have the kitchen cut a large portion in half and put the second half immediately into a doggy bag.
- Order your baked potato with butter and sour cream on the side.
- Order your salad with the dressing on the side.
- Trim the visible chunks of fat from your steak before you eat it.

I did some investigating and came up with the nutrition information for some typical steakhouse menu items. The actual nutrition content of your particular steakhouse item might be higher in fat and calories, but the following information will get you in the ballpark.

Entrées

- **Grilled chicken:** 1 g carbohydrate, 2 g fat (15 percent of calories from fat), 25 g protein, 120 calories.
- **Grilled chicken sandwich**: 39 g carbohydrate, 4 g fat (11 percent of calories from fat), 33 g protein, 324 calories.
- **Grilled salmon (4 oz.):** 1 g carbohydrate, 10 g fat (42 percent of calories from fat), 34 g protein, 240 calories.
- **Sirloin tips with peppers and onions:** 4 g carbohydrate, 8 g fat (35 percent of calories from fat) 27 g protein, 203 calories.
- **Spicy BBQ chicken sandwich:** 45 g carbohydrate, 5 g fat (12 percent of calories from fat), 34 g protein, 368 calories.
- **Home-style chicken fillet:** 21 g carbohydrate, 9 g fat (37 percent of calories from fat), 13 g protein, 217 calories.
- **Junior sirloin steak:** 0 g carbohydrate, 10 g fat (46 percent of calories from fat), 25 g protein, 194 calories.
- **Filet mignon (5.5 oz. cooked):** 0 g carbohydrate, 15 g fat (44 percent of calories from fat), 44 g protein, 0 fiber, 330 calories.
- **Smothered steak sandwich:** 36 g carbohydrate, 15 g fat (31 percent of calories from fat), 34 g protein, 430 calories.
- **Sirloin steak:** 0 g carbohydrate, 16 g fat (51 percent of calories from fat), 34 g protein, 285 calories.
- **Country steak with gravy:** 44 g carbohydrate, 25 g fat (42 percent of calories from fat), 32 g protein, 530 calories.

Sides

- **Baked potato, plain:** 31 g carbohydrate, 0 g fat, 3 g protein, 3 g fiber, 130 calories.

- **Broccoli spears:** 5 g carbohydrate, 0 g fat, 33 g protein, 3 g fiber, 35 calories.

- **Corn (4 oz.):** 28 g carbohydrate, 1.5 g fat (9 percent of calories from fat), 4 g protein, 3 g fat, 120 calories.

- **BBQ beans (4 oz.):** 25 g carbohydrate, 2 g fat (14 percent of calories from fat), 6 g protein, 5 g fiber, 150 calories.

- **Rice pilaf (half cup):** 23 g carbohydrate, 3.5 g fat (23 percent of calories from fat), 2 g protein, 0.5 g fiber, 135 calories.

- **Dinner roll (1):** 14 g carbohydrate, 2 g fat (22 percent of calories from fat), 2 g protein, 1 g fiber, 85 calories.

- **Cornbread (1 piece):** 28 g carbohydrate, 5 g fat (26 percent of calories from fat), 4.5 g protein, 1.5 g fiber, 175 calories.

- **Cinnamon apples:** 34 g carbohydrate, 5 g fat (26 percent of calories from fat), 0 g protein, 2 g fiber, 172 calories.

- **Mashed potatoes (half cup):** 18 g carbohydrate, 5 g fat (35 percent of calories from fat), 2 g protein, 2 g fiber, 115 calories.

- **Biscuit (1):** 29 g carbohydrate, 15 g fat (50 percent of calories from fat), 5 g protein, 1 g fiber, 270 calories.

Soups (1 cup)

- **Vegetable beef:** 18 g carbohydrate, 2 g fat (15 percent of calories from fat), 7 g protein, 3 g fiber, 120 calories.

- **Clam chowder, New England:** 17 g carbohydrate, 9 g fat (45 percent of calories from fat), 3 g protein, 1.5 g fiber, 180 calories.

- **Chili with beans:** 25 g carbohydrates, 9 g fat (30 percent of calories from fat), 23 g protein, 5 g fiber, 270 calories.

Good choices at pizza parlors

Some pizza chains have higher-fat pizza crust, whereas others have the more traditional, bread-type crust. I trust you can tell the difference. But in case you can't, lay your slice of pizza on a thick napkin. Do the grease spots form a triangle where the crust was? The grease from the crust is an indication of its fat content. It's best to frequent the pizza places that have the more traditional bread crusts—that's half the battle. Domino's, for example, makes a hand-tossed pizza crust and a pan crust. The hand tossed is the one you want to ask for, because it has half the fat and saturated fat of a deep-dish pizza.

The second factor in choosing the healthier pizza pie is the toppings—the cheese and all the trimmings. If you ask them to make the pizza with less cheese, this will definitely help. I know you might feel silly doing this, but many of these restaurants really do put on more cheese than pizza really needs. If you are used to the typical sausage and pepperoni pizza, this next tip could be a tough one. If you top your pizza with items that don't add fat calories, but instead add nutrition and fiber—you are hitting the nutrition jackpot. People usually don't have any vegetables with their pizza meal (unless they order a salad), so why not top your pizza with the vegetables you like and make it a more complete meal? Hopefully you like a couple of the following vegetable toppings: peppers, onions, mushrooms, zucchini, fresh tomatoes, broccoli, artichoke hearts, and even fruits such as pineapple. The leaner meat toppings are Canadian bacon and ham.

Blood sugar beware

Pizza seems to be one of those foods that raises blood sugar beyond what the grams of carbohydrates could explain. You might find you tolerate your pizza better if you have a side salad, heavy on the kidney beans, before you eat your pizza. This is probably not a good time to be eating a big slice of cake either. Try two large slices of cheese pizza and see how your blood sugar fares. Two slices will bring you to about 45 g of carbohydrate, 10 g of fat, 13 g of protein, 317 calories, and 669 mg sodium. Two deep-dish slices bring you to 54 g of carbohydrate, 20 g of fat, 18 g of protein, 455 calories, and 1030 mg of sodium.

Bagel shops

I love fresh bagels! Spread with light cream cheese and topped with smoked salmon, they are one of my favorite breakfasts. Bagels look innocent enough, but they can be trouble for some people with diabetes. There's something about those 40-ish grams of carbohydrates that seems to make normal blood sugar difficult first thing in the morning for many people with type 2 diabetes. But there are a few things you can do to try to improve your post-bagel blood sugar.

Try whole-grain bagels or oat-bran bagels to see if that makes a difference. And make sure you balance your mostly carbohydrate bagel with some protein and a little fat. You can do this by spreading your bagel with light cream cheese or filling a savory bagel with some reduced-fat cheese and a slice of turkey breast. Here is how some of these options add up.

- **Whole-grain/wheat bagel with one ounce reduced-fat cheese and one ounce roasted turkey breast:** 55 g carbohydrate, 8 g fat, 23 g protein, 9 g fiber, 375 calories, 842 mg sodium, 30 mg cholesterol.

- **Whole-grain/wheat bagel with two tablespoons light cream cheese:** 54 g carbohydrate, 5.5 g fat, 14 g protein, 9 g fiber, 313 calories, 583 mg sodium, 13 mg cholesterol.

- **Whole-grain/wheat bagel with two tablespoons light cream cheese and one ounce lox or smoked salmon:** 54 g carbohydrate, 6.5 g fat, 19 g protein, 9 g fiber, 346 calories, 1143 mg sodium, 20 mg cholesterol.

- **Whole-grain/wheat bagel with two tablespoons natural style peanut butter:** 59 g carbohydrate, 17 g fat, 18 g protein, 11 g fiber, 460 calories, 570 mg sodium, 0 mg cholesterol.

- **Whole-grain/wheat bagel with one-fourth cup of hummus:** 60 g carbohydrate, 7.5 g fat, 16 g protein, 13 g fiber, 364 calories, 686 mg sodium, 0 mg cholesterol.

Good choices at sandwich shops

There are some really great choices at some sandwich restaurants. If you opt for the whole- or part-wheat selections, your grams of fiber might go up about two to four grams per sandwich. If you add mayonnaise or salad dressing, you'll need to add this into the equation. Good news though: Subway offers light mayonnaise. Other condiments available upon request are mustard, vinegar, and an olive oil blend. Here are some of the best options at Subway (but many of the same options are available at other sandwich chains).

Subway

Salads (doesn't include dressing).

Note: You might want to BYOD (bring your own dressing) because their choices are limited to a higher calorie and fat ranch dressing or a fat free Italian dressing.

- **Veggie Delite Salad:** with 60 calories, 0 g saturated fat, 1 g total fat, 75 mg sodium. Nutrition: 10 g carbs, 3 g protein, 4 g fiber.

- **Oven Roasted Chicken Salad:** 140 calories, 0.5 g saturated fat, 2.5 g total fat, 280 mg sodium. Nutrition: 10 g carbs, 19 g protein, 4 g fiber.

- **Turkey Breast Salad:** 110 calories, 0.5 g saturated fat, 2 g total fat, 580 mg sodium. Nutrition: 12 g carbs, 12 g protein, 4 g fiber.

6-inch sandwiches (made with 9-grain wheat bread, lettuce, tomato, onion, green peppers and cucumbers).

Note: The condiments that add a minimum of calories and sodium are the honey mustard, yellow and Deli brown mustard, olive oil blend, and sweet onion sauce. The vegetables that add nutrition value include spinach, avocado, assorted peppers, lettuce, tomato, and cucumbers.

- **Veggie Delite:** 230 calories, 0.5 g saturated fats, 2.5 g total fat, 310 mg sodium. Nutrition: 44 g carbs, 8 g protein, 5 g fiber.

- **Turkey Breast:** 280 calories, 1 g saturated fat, 3.5 g total fat, 810 mg sodium. Nutrition: 46 g carbs, 18 g protein, 5 g fiber.

- **Turkey Breast with Avocado and Spinach:** 340 calories, 1.5 g saturated fats. 9 g total fat, 790 mg sodium. Nutrition: 49 g carbs, 19 g protein, 8 g fiber.

- **Sweet Onion Chicken Teriyaki:** 380 calories, 1 g saturated fat, 4.5 g total fat, 900 mg sodium. Nutrition: 59 g carbs, 26 g protein, 5 g fiber.

- **Oven Roasted Chicken:** 320 calories, 1.5 g saturated fat, 5 g total fat, 640 mg sodium. Nutrition: 47 g carbs, 23 g protein, 5 g fiber.

- **Roast Beef:** 320 calories, 1.5 g saturated fat, 5 g total fat, 700 mg sodium. Nutrition: 45 g carbs, 24 g protein, 5 g fiber.

- **Steak and Cheese:** 380 calories, 4.5 g saturated fat, 10 g total fat, 1060 mg sodium. Nutrition: 48 g carbs, 26 g protein, 5 g fiber.

Breakfast

- **Egg and Cheese Muffin Melt:** 170 calories, 2 g saturated fat, 6 g total fat, 460 mg sodium. Nutrition: 24 g carbs, 12 g protein, 6 g fiber.

- **Steak, Egg, and Cheese Muffin Melt:** 200 calories, 2.5 g saturated fat, 6 g total fat, 590 mg sodium. Nutrition: 25 g carbs, 15 g protein, 6 g fiber.

- **Egg White and Cheese Muffin Melt:** 150 calories, 1.5 g saturated fat, 3.5 g total fat, 480 mg sodium. Nutrition: 24 g carbs, 12 g protein, 5 g fiber.

- **Egg White with Cheese and Avocado:** 190 calories, 2 g saturated fat, 7 g total fat, 490 mg sodium. Nutrition: 25 g carbs, 12 g protein, 6 g fiber.

Best and worst fast-food breakfasts

The results from a recent University of Minnesota study that noted breakfast habits and weight changes in 2,200 teens over a five-year period, indicated that regular breakfast eaters tended to have the lowest body mass indexes (BMIs) in a dose-response manner. In other words, as breakfast skipping frequency went up, so did the body mass indexes of these teens.

Eating breakfast is definitely good, but if you do end up eating your breakfast at a fast-food chain, remember there are more healthful foods to be had.

In general, "studies show that some people tend to consume more calories, fat, and sodium, and fewer vitamins, on the days when they go to fast-food restaurants than on the days they don't," says Karen Collins, MS, RD, CDN, of the American Institute for Cancer Research.

One reason for this, she says, may be because our bodies don't automatically sense that we need smaller portions when we eat foods high in calories. "Not everyone is able to compensate by eating less later in the day," explains Collins.

In search of a better breakfast

Of course, some fast-food offerings are better than others. Finding a healthier breakfast means looking for items with some fiber and protein (which makes them more satisfying), but not too much saturated fat or total fat. Fiber is important for baked offerings too; even when these items are relatively low in fat, they can be high in sugar and white flour.

A look at the nutrition information that some popular fast-food chains provide on their Websites shows that few of their breakfast items fit the bill. Some offer one or two items that are reasonably low in fat and saturated fat and contain some protein, but they're usually lacking in fiber. Others don't even have one breakfast entree that's low enough in fat and saturated fat to be considered healthy. At Carl's Jr., for example, there was only one main-dish item with less than 20 grams of fat per serving (the French Toast Dips with 18 grams of fat and 2.5 grams of saturated fat). It does contribute nine grams of protein, but is lacking in the fiber department, with only one gram. Their worst choice on the breakfast menu is the Carl's Jr. Loaded Breakfast Burrito with 820 calories, 51 grams of fat, 16 grams of saturated fat, 595 milligrams of cholesterol, and 1530 milligrams of sodium.

No matter which fast-food chain you visit, though, high-fat and high-calorie breakfast choices abound. When you find yourself at a fast-food or quick-serve chain before 11 a.m., choose a better breakfast option, keep your portions reasonable, and keep (or start!) exercising.

Best breakfast choices at each fast-food chain

- **Apple Cinnamon Walnut Oatmeal (McDonald's):** 270 calories, 8 g fat, 2 g saturated fat, 5 mg cholesterol, 105 mg sodium, 5 g fiber, 45 g carbohydrate, 6 g protein.

- **Multigrain Oatmeal with mixed nuts and dried fruit (Chick-fil-A):** 290 calories, 11 g fat, 1 g saturated fat, 0 mg cholesterol, 70 mg sodium, 6 grams fiber, 50 g carbohydrate, 2 g protein.

- **Quaker Oatmeal Original (Burger King):** 140 calories, 3.5 g fat, 1 g saturated fat, 5 mg cholesterol, 100 mg sodium, 3 g fiber, 23 g carbohydrate, 5 g protein.

- **Yogurt Parfait with granola (Chick-fil-A):** 290 calories, 6 g fat, 2 g saturated fat, 10 mg cholesterol, 85 mg sodium, 1 g fiber, 53 g carbohydrate, 7 g protein.

- **Breakfast Jack (Jack in the Box):** 283 calories, 11 g fat, 4 g saturated fat, 239 mg cholesterol, 780 mg sodium, 1 g fiber, 30 g carbohydrate, 16 g protein.

- **Egg McMuffin (McDonald's):** 300 calories, 12 g fat, 5 g saturated fat, 260 mg cholesterol, 780 mg sodium, 2 g fiber, 30 g carbohydrate, 18 g protein.

- **Breakfast Muffin Sandwich Egg and Cheese (Burger King):** 260 calories, 11 g fat, 4 g saturated fat, 170 mg cholesterol, 830 mg sodium, 2 g fiber, 27 g carbohydrate, 13 g protein.

Chapter 8
Smart Snacking and Balanced Breakfasts

There are two specific areas of eating that Certified Diabetes Educators wanted me to give some extra information about—smart snacking and eating balanced breakfasts. So with all the information in this book behind you, here are two final ways you can help bring on better blood sugar.

Smart snacking

Do the words *chips*, *cookies*, *ice cream*, *candy bars*, or *crackers* mean anything to you? These high-calorie, fatty, or sugary foods represent our more popular snack foods. But to start snacking wisely, you don't necessarily need to trade all your Chips Ahoy cookies for carrot sticks, or your carton of ice cream for a carton of tofu. We can make smarter snack choices by choosing whole foods or foods that are higher in fiber and important nutrients, that feature carbohydrates with lower glycemic indexes, and that are balanced with some protein and some of the more heart-helpful fats.

Some people with diabetes need to eat snacks to help prevent low blood glucose levels (mostly people with type 1 diabetes). These healthful snacks can be eaten before going to bed, before exercising, or at other times when hypoglycemia tends to strike. For the people with diabetes who are more at risk of having high blood sugar (hyperglycemia), which is most people with type 2 diabetes, smart snacks would include higher-fiber, lower-glycemic index ingredients.

Soluble fiber snacks

Foods rich in soluble fiber make for great snacks because soluble fiber leaves the stomach slowly, encouraging better blood sugar and making you feel satisfied longer. Here are some possible snack ingredients that are high in soluble fiber:

- **Peas and beans:** These include canned vegetarian or fat-free refried beans, green salad with canned kidney beans added, three-bean salad made with a light vinaigrette salad dressing.
- **Oats and oat bran:** Examples are low-sugar hot oatmeal, low-sugar oat or oat-bran muffin, or low-sugar oat breakfast cereal.
- **Barley:** It can be found in barley added to vegetable soup or stew.
- **Some fruits:** Fruits such as apples, peaches, citrus fruits, mango, plums, kiwis, pears, and berries can be blended in a smoothie, enjoyed with a whole-grain low-sugar cereal, or mixed in plain or light yogurt.
- **Some vegetables:** These include artichokes, celery root, sweet potatoes, parsnips, turnips, acorn squash, Brussels sprouts, cabbage, green peas, broccoli, carrots, cauliflower, asparagus, and beets.

Adding other plant foods that contribute some smart fat and/or protein into our snack recipes, such as nuts, soy foods, olive and canola oil, and avocado, may also help minimize high blood sugar resulting from traditionally high-carbohydrate snacks.

To help you practice smarter snacking and encourage better blood sugar, here are six more tips and recipes!

1. Whole-grain snacks are a step in the right direction.

The latest research suggests that people who eat whole grains have the lowest incidence of diabetes. They appear to increase the efficiency of insulin so that less is required to metabolize the sugar.

After speaking with a few bagel-lovers, I thought I would calculate how to make a better bagel snack. Bagels are mostly carbohydrates, so it is important to top them with something that will add some protein and fat into the snack equation. This will make the bagel more satisfying, and the energy will hit the bloodstream more slowly and last longer. This topping could be a little bit of natural-style peanut butter, some light cream cheese, or a slice of reduced-fat cheese and a slice of turkey breast.

The other key to a better bagel snack is eating whole wheat or whole grain. This will pump some fiber into the picture. Whole grains also contribute vitamin and minerals and phytochemicals that you aren't getting in bagels made with refined flour.

Bagel and Cream Cheese

Makes one bagel snack.

1/2 whole wheat or whole grain bagel, toasted or untoasted.
1 Tbs. of light cream cheese.

Per serving: 108 calories, 2.7 g fiber, 4.5 g protein, 16.5 g carbohydrate, 2.9 g fat, 1.8 g saturated fat, 7.5 mg cholesterol, 210 mg sodium. Calories from fat: 24 percent.

2. Some foods do not cause high blood sugar.

Even in large amounts, if eaten alone, the following foods are not likely to result in a substantial rise in blood sugar:

- Meat.
- Poultry.
- Fish.
- Avocados.
- Salad vegetables.
- Cheese.
- Eggs.

(Foster-Powell et al., "International table of glycemic index and glycemic load values." *Am J Clin Nutr* 76 [2002]: 5–56.)

Mini Turkey Melts

This snack works well with the toaster oven.
Makes two snack servings.
10 Triscuits.
5 thin slices of turkey breast cut in half.
2 oz. shredded, reduced-fat cheese of choice (Jarlsberg Lite, cheddar, jack).
1/4 avocado, cut into bite-size pieces (optional).

1. Place 10 Triscuits in a toaster oven pan. Top each with half a slice of turkey (fold it over to fit).
2. Top the turkey with shredded cheese.
3. Broil in toaster oven, watching carefully, until cheese is nicely melted.
4. Top each cracker with a piece of avocado, if desired, and enjoy!

Per serving: 214 calories, 21 g protein, 16 g carbohydrate, 7 g fat (3.5 g saturated fat, 2.2 g monounsaturated fat, .1 g polyunsaturated fat), 40 mg cholesterol,

2 g fiber, 260 mg sodium (not including the sodium from the turkey; the sodium in turkey slices vary greatly by brand). Calories from fat: 29 percent.

3. Low glycemic index foods are less refined.

Low glycemic index foods are generally less refined than their higher glycemic index counterparts. For example, white bread has a glycemic index of 105 and a glycemic load of 10, whereas Healthy Choice Hearty 7 Grain bread has a glycemic index of 79 and a glycemic load of 8. Corn flakes have a glycemic index of 130 and a glycemic load of 24, whereas Raisin Bran cereal has a glycemic index of 87 (plus or minus 7) and a glycemic load of 12.

Quick Vegetable Bean Salad

One serving of this quick salad gives you a dose of alpha- and beta-carotene, folic acid, vitamin C, fiber (and plant omega-3 fatty acids from the canola oil). If you want to make this more of a meal, stir in a can of albacore tuna to add fish omega-3 fatty acids and some protein into the picture.

Makes eight servings.

3 cups baby carrots, or diced or thinly sliced carrots.

3 cups broccoli florets cut into bite-size pieces.

1 15-oz. can kidney beans, rinsed and drained well.

1/2 cup finely chopped mild onion (use less if desired).

1/2 cup "1/3 less fat" bottled vinaigrette made with canola or olive oil. (I use Seven Seas 1/3 less fat Red Wine Vinaigrette with canola.)

1 6-oz. can albacore tuna in water (optional).

1. Combine the carrot pieces with 1/4 cup water in a microwave-safe covered dish and cook on high for about three to five minutes (or until just barely tender). Drain well and add to medium-sized serving bowl.

2. Combine the broccoli pieces with 1/4 cup water in a microwave-safe covered dish and cook on high for about three to five minutes (or until just barely tender). Drain well and add to medium-sized serving bowl.

3. Add beans, chopped onion, and vinaigrette (and tuna if desired) to serving bowl. Toss well to blend.

Per serving: 110 calories, 5 g protein, 19 g carbohydrate, 2.5 g fat, 0 g saturated fat, 0 mg cholesterol, 7 g fiber, 310 mg sodium. Calories from fat: 20 percent.

4. Go ahead, get nutty.

An ounce of most nuts will add about 170 calories (with around seven grams carbohydrate, six grams protein, and 15 grams fat). Which nuts are best? Hazelnuts and almonds are lowest in saturated fat, with macadamia and hazelnuts being the highest in monounsaturated fat (this is a good thing). Pistachios and macadamia nuts were highest in fiber (about three grams per ounce) with walnuts scoring highest in omega-3 fatty acids. So bottom line: They are all good!

Peanut Butter Banana Fana

Makes two snack servings.

1 banana.
2 Tbs. smooth natural-style peanut butter
Topping to roll banana in, such as Rice Krispies cereal, granola, or Grapenuts.

1. Peel banana. Place on piece of foil and freeze for one hour. Meanwhile, remove peanut butter from refrigerator and bring to room temperature (so it's more spreadable).
2. Using a dinner knife, spread the peanut butter all around the banana.
3. Roll in food topping of choice, such as 1/2 cup of Rice Krispies cereal.
4. Place on foil sheet and refrigerate for one hour. It's ready to eat!

Per serving (with Rice Krispies cereal): 175 calories, 5.5 g protein, 22 g carbohydrate, 8 g fat, 1 g saturated fat, 0 mg cholesterol, 2.4 g fiber, 55 mg sodium. Calories from fat: 42 percent.

5. Yodel for Greek yogurt.

I am a Greek yogurt fan and have some almost every day in my smoothies or as a fruit parfait. It makes a great snack because it contributes important nutrients and along with the carbohydrates (about 23 grams in 6 oz. of nonfat vanilla Greek yogurt) you get 11 grams of protein. Enjoy yogurt with fruit and a high fiber cereal or nuts, or it can be the creamy ingredient in your smoothie.

Mini Yogurt Parfait

Yogurt makes a great snack, but day after day it can get a bit boring. One way to make it a little more interesting is to make a parfait with layers of yogurt, fresh or frozen fruit, and low-fat granola. Here's one way to do this.

Makes one parfait.

Layer half of each of the following ingredients in a parfait glass, and then repeat with the other half.

1/4 cup fresh fruit (such as berries or sliced peaches).

1/2 cup nonfat plain Greek yogurt (4 ounces).

1/4 cup low-fat granola (other high-fiber cereal or nuts can be substituted).

Per parfait: 186 calories, 15 g protein, 30 g carbohydrates, 2 g fat, .3 g saturated fat, 0 mg cholesterol, 4 g fiber, 111 mg sodium, 125 mg calcium. Calories from fat: 10 percent.

6. Enjoy portable fruit.

Fruit can travel well in your car or briefcase and comes in handy for a quick pick-me-up. Many fruits offer just enough carbohydrates with a nice dose of fiber. The following fruits have a low glycemic load (five or less per serving):

- Cherries, glycemic load of 3 per (4 1/4 ounce) serving.

- Grapefruit, glycemic load of 3 per (4 1/4 ounce) serving.

- Kiwi fruit, glycemic load of 5 per (4 1/4 ounce) serving.

- Oranges, glycemic load of 5 per (4 1/4 ounce) serving.

- Peaches (fresh or canned in juice), glycemic load of 4 per (4 1/4 ounce) serving.

- Pears, glycemic load of 4 per (4 1/4 ounce) serving.

- Plums, glycemic load of 3 per (4 1/4 ounce) serving.

- Cantaloupe, glycemic load of 4 per (4 1/4 ounce) serving.

- Strawberries, glycemic load of 1 per (4 1/4 ounce) serving

Melon Medley

Chilled melon is a refreshing afternoon or evening snack. Make a bowl of melon cubes or balls, cover the bowl, and keep it in the refrigerator for a quick snack.

Dessert tip: turn this into a dessert by topping 1/2 cup light vanilla ice cream or frozen Greek yogurt with the chopped melon, and then drizzle a little honey over the top!

Makes four snack servings.

3 cups honeydew melon balls or cubes.

3 cups cantaloupe balls or cubes.

In serving bowl, toss melon to mix.

Per serving: 87 calories, 1.6 g protein, 21.8 g carbohydrates, 0.5 g fat, 0 g saturated fat, 0 mg cholesterol, 1.7 g fiber, 23 mg sodium. Calories from fat: 4 percent.

Other snack suggestions

Pear and Jarlsberg Lite

This is one of my favorite snacks—pairing pear wedges with a nicely flavored cheese such as Jarlsberg Lite or Gruyere. What a great way to work another fruit serving into my day!

Per serving (1 sliced pear with 1 ounce of sliced Jarlsberg Lite): 202 calories, 9 grams protein, 32.5 g carbohydrate, 5.5 g fat (3 g saturated fat, 1.6 g monounsaturated fat, 0.3 g polyunsaturated fat), 15 mg cholesterol, 5 g fiber, 150 mg sodium, Calories from fat: 24 percent.

Healthy Pop Jolly Time popcorn

You knew it was coming. Sooner or later I would have to list microwave popcorn as a snack! Some of the microwave popcorn companies are still using partially hydrogenated oils in some of their products, which means that some of their products have trans fats. They tend to be in the "movie theatre" or "butter" flavors.

All you need is a popcorn packet and a microwave—at home, at work, or even at the swim club—and you are good to go.

There are a few brands with a 94-percent fat free (or thereabouts) microwave popping corn. I'm going to give you the nutritional analysis for Jolly Time's Healthy Pop Butter Flavor Microwave Pop Corn.

Per serving (5 cups popped—about 2 1/2 servings per bag): 90 calories, 2 g fat, 2 g saturated fat, 0 mg cholesterol, 210 mg sodium, 23 g carb, 9 g dietary fiber, and 4 g protein.

Wendy's Side Salad

I found myself in the Wendy's drive through recently ordering side salads for me and my girls, as we were rushing to the orthodontist and all in need of an afternoon snack. It's actually a fresh and colorful salad, and, best of all, it's on the 99-cents menu!

Per serving (side salad and dressed with half a packet—2.5 ounces total—of reduced-fat creamy ranch dressing): 90 calories, 10.5 g carbohydrate, 2.5 g protein, 4.5 g fat, 0.7 g saturated fat, 7 mg cholesterol, about 2.5 g fiber, and 325 mg sodium.

Balanced breakfasts

If you normally eat dinner at 7 p.m., breakfast the next day is the first food your body has had in about 11 hours. When we put it that way, breakfast sure sounds important to the body's functioning, doesn't it?

It's better, health-wise, to eat breakfast than to not eat breakfast, but it's definitely best to eat a balanced, nutrient-rich, higher fiber breakfast than one that is full of refined grains, sugar, salt and/or saturated fat, whether or not you have type 2 diabetes!

To eat breakfast or not eat breakfast? That is the question.

Some people may think skipping breakfast is a good way to trim calories and lose weight, but recent studies suggest the exact opposite. New research suggests the daily act of eating breakfast may decrease our risk of obesity, even after researchers controlled for other dietary factors and physical activity.

To maintain good health and prevent those hard-to-lose pounds from creeping on in the first place, make it a habit to eat a balanced breakfast. Many people go wrong by eating a breakfast with mostly refined carbohydrates and very little fiber and protein—such as a refined flour bagel or a muffin made with sugar and white flour, or a sugary, low-fiber breakfast cereal. For a more satisfying meal, balancing carbohydrates (preferably from whole grains, fruits, and vegetables) with some protein and a little smart fat will do a better job of staving off hunger until lunch and fueling your entire morning's activities. Making sure to have a protein-rich breakfast may also decrease your susceptibility to choose or snack on junk-type "reward" foods later in the day, according to a recent study with overweight teenage girls (although more research needs to be done to clarify this finding). (*Obesity, Silver Spring* 19(10) [October 2011]: 2019–25.)

What is your best breakfast if your blood sugar tends to be high in the morning?

What kinds of breakfasts are best for people with type 2 diabetes?

Step 1: It's best to *have* breakfast.

Skipping breakfast can put a strain on your body by continuing the state of fasting. And, according to this new research with male health professionals aged 45 to 82, it may even lead to risk factors including obesity, high blood pressure and diabetes (*Circulation*, 128, no. 4, 337–343).

So, given it is best for your body to not skip breakfast, what is a better breakfast if you have type 2 diabetes and your blood sugar tends to be high in the morning?

Step 2: Fix a balanced breakfast!

Many people tend to be more resistant to insulin in the morning, which means that carbohydrates may be less tolerated at breakfast than at other meals. Start by fixing a balanced breakfast that includes some protein plus some smart carbohydrates (not processed) and smart fats (such as nuts, avocado, extra virgin olive oil, and almond or soy milk).

Breakfasts that have fiber, protein, and slowly digested carbohydrates are best because they are more likely to energize your entire morning and stave off hunger. Here are some examples of quick and easy, yet satisfying breakfasts:

- Hot oatmeal made with soy or low fat milk, with some fresh or frozen berries and a sprinkle of nuts.

- Cold whole-grain, high-fiber cereal with added nuts and soy, almond or cow's milk, fresh or frozen berries.

- French toast made with whole-wheat bread, topped with some fresh fruit. You can make the French toast on the weekend and freeze the leftovers for a busy weekday morning. Just pop it in the microwave to warm it up.

- A scrambled egg with two egg whites, with spinach, fresh tomatoes, and avocado, served with whole-wheat toast, can be made in about five minutes. Add a sprinkle of cheese if desired.

- Nonfat Greek yogurt typically contains two times the protein of regular yogurt. Top it with fresh or frozen berries and some high-fiber granola or nuts.

- Buckwheat or whole-grain pancakes with lean chicken or turkey (or soy-based) sausages and 1/2 cup of fresh or frozen fruit.

- Greek yogurt smoothie made with 1/2 cup nonfat vanilla Greek yogurt, 1 to 1 1/2 cups fresh or frozen fruit, 1/3 cup low-fat milk or soy or almond milk.

- Whole grain bagel or English muffin or two slices of whole-wheat toast with natural style peanut butter, a scrambled egg, hummus, light cream cheese, and smoked salmon, or part-skim cheese.

Strive for at least 15 grams of protein

One quick tip I use to keep my breakfast balanced is to "strive for 15!" I try to include five to 10 grams of fiber and 15 grams of protein in every breakfast.

Lower fat or nonfat dairy products will add protein to your breakfast, along with eggs, egg white or egg substitute, lean breakfast meat options (Canadian bacon or extra lean ham, turkey bacon, light turkey sausage), and soy milk and soy products.

Breakfast Protein Options

Protein Options	Protein (g)	Calories	Fat (g)	Sat. Fat (g)	Carbs (g)
skim milk, 1 cup	10	100	0	0	14
low-fat yogurt, vanilla, 1 cup	9.3	253	4.6	2.6	42
low-fat cottage cheese, 1 cup	28	160	2	1	6
reduced-fat Cheese, 1 ounce	8	70	4	2.5	1
egg whites, 2	7	33	0	0	1
egg substitute, 1/4 cup		6	30	0	0
soy milk, low-fat, 1 cup	4	90	1.5	0	14
soy-based sausage, 2 ounces	12	119	4.5	0.7	6
tofu, extra firm, light, 2 ounces	5	43	1.4	0	2.2
Canadian bacon, 2 ounces	12	89	3.9	1.2	1
extra-lean ham, 2 ounces	11	61	1.5	0.4	0.4
turkey bacon, 2 strips	4	70	6	2	1
light turkey sausage, 2 ounces	9	130	10	2.2	1
peanut butter, natural, 2 tablespoons	7	200	16	2	7
light cream cheese, 1 ounce	3	53	4	2.7	1.8
lox (smoked salmon), 1 ounce	5.2	33	1.2	0.2	0

Try for 10 grams of fiber

One way to get closer to those 10 grams of fiber is to include a whole grain and/or fruits or vegetables with breakfast. I look for opportunities to switch to whole grains, because of the plethora of health benefits they offer, and breakfast is the perfect time to work in a serving or two. Whole grains offer a myriad of vitamins, minerals, and phytochemicals that, together, are likely to have significant health benefits beyond the fiber. New research suggests that eating whole grains may help reduce your risk of cardiovascular disease and certain cancers, as well as developing type 2 diabetes by improving insulin sensitivity, improving serum lipid levels, and lowering oxidative stress.

Get your grains at breakfast by choosing from the following:

- Hot oatmeal (or another hot whole-grain cereal).

- Cold whole-grain cereal.

- 100-percent whole-wheat bread/toast, small bagel or English muffin, or tortilla.

- Pancakes and waffles made with at least half whole-wheat flour plus oats, oat bran, or ground flaxseed added sometimes as well.

- Muffins and cinnamon rolls made with at least half whole-wheat flour plus oats, oat bran or ground flaxseed added sometimes as well.

Weekend breakfast tip

If you have extra whole grain waffles, pancakes, muffins, and so on from the weekend, just freeze them in individual plastic bags for part of a quick breakfast during the week. Just pop them from the freezer into the microwave or toaster/toaster oven.

Other foods that help add fiber come from the plant food groups; fruits, vegetables, other whole grains, beans, and nuts.

Possible Options	Fiber (g)	Calories	Carbs (g)	Fat (g)	Protein (g)
Grains:					
oatmeal, cooked, 3/4 cup	3	124	21	2.7	4.5
whole-grain cereal, 1 cup	7	190	45	1.5	5
whole-wheat bread, 1	2	70	14	1	3
whole-wheat bagel (95 g)	9	260	52	1.5	11
whole-wheat tortilla (114 g)	8	300	54	4.5	12

Possible Options	Fiber (g)	Calories	Carbs (g)	Fat (g)	Protein (g)
whole-wheat flour, 1/4 cup	4	110	23	0.5	4
oats, rolled, quick, 1/4 cup	2.3	83	14	1.5	3
barley, med, cooked, 1/2 cup	5	220	55	0.7	5
barley, pearl, cooked, 1/2 cup	3	97	22	0.3	2
buckwheat groats, cooked, 1/2 cup	2.3	77	17	0.5	2.8
quinoa, cooked, 1/2 cup	2.6	111	20	1.8	4
Fruit:					
banana, 1	3.1	105	27	0.4	1.3
blueberries, fresh, 1/2 cup	2	42	11	0.2	0.6
raspberries, fresh, 1/2 cup	4	32	7	0.4	0.7
dried fruit, mixed, 1/4 cup	2	120	28	0	1
melon, 2 cups (cantaloupe or honeydew)	3	108	26	0.3	3
Possible Options	**Fiber (g)**	**Calories**	**Carbs (g)**	**Fat (g)**	**Protein (g)**
Vegetables:					
mushrooms, cooked, 1/2 cup	2	22	4	0.4	2
onions, cooked, 1/2 cup	2	29	7	0.1	1

zucchini, cooked, 1 cup	2.2	26	5	0.2	2
tomatoes, 1 med.	1	25	5	0	1
Nuts and seeds:					
ground flaxseed, 2 Tbs.	3	80	4	6	3
pecans (or chopped nuts), 1/4 cup	3	205	4	21	3

Seven balanced breakfast examples with 50 grams of carbohydrate, or fewer!

1. Omelet made with 1/2 cup egg substitute, 1/2 cup vegetables, 1 ounce reduced-fat cheese served on 100-percent whole grain English muffin (288 calories, **35 g carbohydrate**, 7 g fiber, 28 g protein, 6 g fat, 2.5 g saturated fat, 15 mg cholesterol, 724 mg sodium).

2. Multigrain waffle topped with 1/2-cup fresh fruit and 1/4-cup Greek plain yogurt, with 1/8 teaspoon vanilla extract and a pinch of ground cinnamon stirred in (265 calories, **48 g carbohydrate**, 8 g fiber, 19 g protein, 5 g fat, 1 g saturated fat, 12 mg cholesterol, 386 mg sodium).

3. Two slices French toast made with whole-grain bread and one higher omega-3 egg blended with 1/4 cup fat-free half-and-half or low-fat milk plus 1/8 teaspoon vanilla and a pinch of ground cinnamon (278 calories, **42 g carbohydrate**, 5 g fiber, 14 g protein, 6.5 g fat, 1.5 g saturated fat, 215 mg cholesterol, 480 mg sodium).

4. Breakfast burrito made with 1 whole wheat tortilla (about 50 grams in weight per tortilla), 1/2 cup egg substitute scrambled with 1/2 cup assorted cooked vegetables, and 1 ounce of reduced-fat cheese (304 calories, **32 g carbohydrate**, 6 g fiber, 25 g protein, 7 g fat, 2.5 g saturated fat, 15 mg cholesterol, 669 mg sodium).

5. Homemade breakfast muffin sandwich made with 1 whole-grain English muffin, 1 1/2-ounces light turkey breakfast sausage, and 1 ounce reduced-fat cheese (300 calories, **28 g carbohydrate**, 5 g fiber, 21 g protein, 12 g fat, 4 g saturated fat, 83 mg cholesterol, 690 mg sodium).

6. Smoothie made with 6 ounces Greek yogurt blended with 1 cup frozen fruit and 1/2-cup soy milk or low-fat milk (230 calories, **42 g carbohydrate**, 6.5 g fiber, 14 g protein, 4 g fat, 1 g saturated fat, 5 mg cholesterol, 130 mg sodium).

7. Yogurt breakfast parfait made with 6 ounces vanilla Greek yogurt, 1/2-cup fresh fruit (such as raspberries), topped with 1/8 cup nuts, such as walnuts, and 1/2 cup whole-grain cereal, such as Grape Nut Flakes (300 calories, **44 g carbohydrate**, 7 g fiber, 15 g protein, 9.3 g fat, 0 g saturated fat, 0 mg cholesterol, 179 mg sodium).

Sources:

Nutritional Analysis by ESHA Research Food Processor SQL.

Smith Edge M. et al. "A New Life for Whole Grains." *Journal of the American Dietetic Association* 105, no. 12 (December 2005): 1856–1860.

Timlin M.T. et al. "Breakfast Eating and Weight Change in a 5-Year Prospective Analysis of Adolescents: Project EAT." *Pediatrics* 121, no. 3 (March 2008): e638–e645.

Bonus breakfast recipes

Strawberry Summer Muffins

These muffins are delicious fresh from the oven. If you are in the habit of spreading butter or margarine on your muffins, try some light cream cheese on these instead.

Makes 11 muffins (5.5 servings of two muffins each).

1 1/3 cup sliced fresh strawberries (frozen can also be used).

1/4 cup low-fat milk.

1 tsp. vanilla extract.

1/2 tsp. strawberry or raspberry extract (optional).

1/2 tsp. red food coloring (optional).

1/4 cup reduced-fat margarine with the least amount of saturated/trans fat (with about 8 grams of fat per Tbs.).

1/2 cup granulated sugar (add 1/4 cup more sugar or Splenda if you prefer it sweeter).

1 large egg, room temperature (higher omega-3 if available).

1/4 cup egg substitute or 2 egg whites.

1 cup whole-wheat flour.

1/2 cup unbleached white flour.

1 tsp. baking powder.

1/4 tsp. salt.

1 Tbs. powdered sugar for dusting the tops (optional).

1. Preheat oven to 350 degrees. Line a 12-cup muffin tin with cupcake liners; set aside. Place strawberries in a small food processor; process until pureed. Make sure you have 2/3 cup of puree.

2. In a small bowl, combine 2/3 cup strawberry puree with low-fat milk, vanilla extract, strawberry extract, and red food coloring (if desired); set aside.

3. In a bowl of an electric mixer fitted with the paddle attachment, cream margarine and sugar on medium-high speed, until combined and fluffy. Reduce speed to medium-low and add the egg and egg substitute or egg white, beating just until blended. Make sure to scrape the side and bottom of bowl well halfway through.

4. With the mixer turned off, in a medium bowl, whisk together flours, baking powder, and salt then add half of the flour mixture to the mixing bowl with margarine mixture, beating just until blended. Pour in the strawberry mixture and beat on low just until blended, scraping the sides of the bowl with spatula midway. Add in the remaining flour mixture, beating just until blended and scraping down sides of the bowl.

5. Add 1/4 cup of muffin batter to each prepared muffin cup. Bake until tops are just dry to the touch (about 22 minutes). Let cool completely in tin before dusting with powdered sugar if desired.

Per two-muffin serving: 258 calories, 8 g protein, 47 g carbohydrate, 6 g fat, 1 g saturated fat, 40 mg cholesterol, 4 g fiber, 260 mg sodium. Calories from fat: 20 percent.

Veggie Microwave Frittata

This is a tasty breakfast dish for two made in about 10 minutes. You can garnish each serving with fresh chopped tomato or salsa and/or avocado wedges.

Makes two servings.

1 1/4 cup shredded fat-free frozen hash browns.

2/3 cup shredded or grated carrot, chopped zucchini, or broccoli.

1/4 cup chopped onion.

1 Tbs. chopped fresh parsley (or 1 1/2 tsp. parsley flakes).

2 tsp. olive oil or canola oil.

Pinch salt and pepper (optional).

2 large eggs (higher omega-3 fatty acids if available).

1/2 cups egg substitute.

1/4 cup low-fat milk or fat-free half-and-half.

1/8 tsp. dry mustard.

2 dashes hot pepper sauce (such as Tabasco).

1/2 cup shredded reduced-fat sharp cheddar cheese.

1. In a microwave-safe 1-quart casserole dish, combine potatoes, carrot, onion, parsley, and oil. Cover and microwave on high for three minutes, stirring after 90 seconds. Add salt and pepper if desired.
2. In a mixing bowl, combine eggs, egg substitute, milk, mustard, and hot pepper sauce by beating on medium speed for a minute or two. Pour egg mixture into casserole dish and stir to combine with potato mixture.
3. Cover dish (waxed paper will work) and microwave on high for two minutes. Draw cooked egg toward the middle of dish and the liquid egg toward the edges and microwave on high for two minutes more. Sprinkle cheese on top and microwave until melted (about 30 seconds more). Let stand a few minutes before serving.

Per serving: 280 calories, 20 g protein, 21 g carbohydrate, 13 g fat, 4.3 g saturated fat, 6.2 g monounsaturated fat, 1.2 g polyunsaturated fat, 218 mg cholesterol, 2.2 g fiber, 296 mg sodium. Calories from fat: 42 percent.

Index

179

About the Author

Elaine Magee is positively passionate about changing the way America eats—one recipe at a time! Her national column, *The Recipe Doctor*, appeared in newspapers such as the *Atlanta Journal-Constitution*, *Democrat and Chronicle*, *Hartford Courant*, *Honolulu Advertiser*, and magazines such as *Today's Health & Wellness* for a decade. In the column she performed recipe "makeovers," in which she was able to bring down the calories, fat, saturated fat, and sometimes sugar and sodium while increasing fiber, phytochemicals, omega-3s, and monounsaturated fat. Elaine is known for "doctoring" real recipes while retaining the original good taste. And she keeps it easy. She believes that if there is a shortcut in the kitchen, you should take it!

Elaine is the author of more than 25 books on nutrition and healthy cooking, including *Food Synergy* (Rodale, March 2008). Elaine's medical nutrition series includes *Tell Me What to Eat If I Have Diabetes*, *Tell Me What to Eat If I Have Irritable Bowel Syndrome*, and *Tell Me What to Eat If I Have Acid Reflux*. Hundreds of thousands of these books have been sold, and they are now being distributed all over the world, including China, Russia, Spain, Indonesia, and the Middle East.

Elaine is currently the wellness and performance nutritionist for Stanford University and continues to consult to Websites and food companies and councils including Web MD (10 years), the Mushroom Council, and more.

Over the years Elaine has contributed thousands of articles and recipes to national magazines and has appeared on national/regional radio and television.

Elaine graduated as the Nutrition Science Department "Student of the Year" from San Jose State University with a bachelor of science in nutrition and a minor in chemistry. She also obtained her master's degree in public health nutrition from UC–Berkeley and is a registered dietitian. She was a nutrition instructor at Diablo Valley College for two years and the nutrition marketing specialist (California Department of Health) for the now national "5 a Day" health program for three years.

Visit Elaine's Website at *www.recipedoctor.com.*

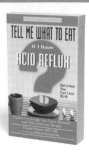
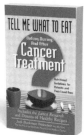
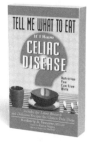
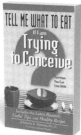

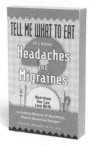
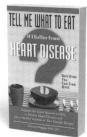
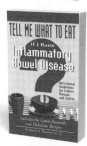
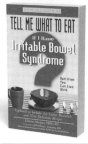